Imaging
of the
Newborn Baby

*To the babies and their families who have both
taught us and trusted us; and to the nursing,
radiographic, medical and other colleagues who
have helped us look after them.*

For Churchill Livingstone:

Commissioning editors: Timothy Horne, Maria Khan
Project editor: Barbara Simmons
Production controller: Nancy Arnott
Design direction: Erik Bigland

Imaging of the Newborn Baby

Edited by

Haresh Kirpalani

BM FRCP(Canada) FRCP(Lond) MSc
Professor, Neonatal and Pediatric Critical Care,
Department of Pediatrics, Children's Hospital,
McMaster University Medical Centre at
Hamilton Health Sciences Corporation,
Ontario, Canada

Gerald Gill

MD MRCP(Canada)
Associate Professor, Department of Pediatric
Radiology, McMaster University Medical
Centre at Hamilton Health Sciences
Corporation, Ontario, Canada

John Mernagh

MD PhD FRCP(Canada)
Assistant Professor, Department of Radiology,
Children's Hospital, McMaster University
Medical Centre at Hamilton Health Sciences
Corporation, Ontario, Canada

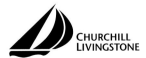

CHURCHILL
LIVINGSTONE

EDINBURGH LONDON NEW YORK PHILADELPHIA SYDNEY TORONTO 1999

CHURCHILL LIVINGSTONE
An imprint of Elsevier Science Limited

First published 1999
  Reprinted 2001, 2002

ISBN 0443 055440

British Library of Cataloguing in Publication Data
A catalogue record for this book is available from the
British Library.

Library of Congress Cataloging in Publication Data
A catalog record for this book is available from the Library
of Congress.

Medical knowledge is constantly changing. As
information becomes available, changes in treatment,
procedures, equipment and the use of drugs become
necessary. The author and publishers have, as far as it is
possible, taken care to ensure that the information given in
this text is accurate and up to date. However, readers are
strongly advised to confirm that the information, especially
with regard to drug usage, complies with current
legislation and standards of practice.

The
publisher's
policy is to use
**paper manufactured
from sustainable forests**

Printed in China by RDC Group Limited
C/03

Foreword

The methods used for and interpretations of radiological evaluations of newborns are quite distinct from general radiology. The sizes of the subjects, risks of procedures and exposures, and the unique diseases of the newborn require selective and cautious use of radiological procedures. This handbook provides a concise yet thorough summary of not only radiological findings in newborns but also an integration of those findings into a clinical context and the pathophysiology of the unique diseases of newborns. The premise for the organization of the book is that a team approach to neonatal radiology is essential for optimal assessments. This message is effectively conveyed by the blending of clinical history with comparisons of various techniques for radiological assessments. The practical suggestions for how best to perform radiological evaluations with clear explanations of limitations and risks will be especially useful for clinicians working with such neonates. This book is a superb teaching manual for those involved in the care of the newborn. Its impact will be most beneficial if all members of the care team take to heart the message that a team approach for selecting, performing and interpreting newborn radiology is most likely to achieve the best outcomes with the lowest risks.

Alan Jobe MD PhD
Professor of Neonatology, Neonatal and Pulmonary Biology, Cincinnati Children's Hospital Medical Centre, Cincinnati, Ohio, USA

Acknowledgements

Contributors

Our thanks are due to Dr Robert Williams of Montreal Children's Hospital for most of the films in the cardiac section; to Dr Andrew Whitelaw of Bristol University for some advice on the brain chapter; to all the staff at McMaster University Neonatal Intensive Care Unit, who vigilantly alerted us to the latest interesting XRs; and importantly – to all the editorial staff (especially Barbara Simmons) whose patient nudging to get it finished was vital.

Pamela Cairns MB BCh MRCP(UK) MRCPCH DCH
Neonatal Fellow, Children's Hospital, McMaster Medical Centre at Hamilton Health Sciences Corporation, Ontario, Canada

Cynthia Cupido MD MSc
Senior Resident, Department of Paediatrics, MacMaster University Medical Centre at Hamilton Health Sciences Corporation, Ontario, Canada

Patrick T. Mohide MD FRCS(C) MSc(DME)
Professor and Chair, Department of Obstetrics and Gynaecology, McMaster University, Ontario Canada

Aideen M. Moore FRCP(C) MRCP(I)
Assistant Professor, Neonatology, Hospital for Sick Children, Toronto, Ontario, Canada

Mark Walton BMed MD FRCS(C)
Associate Professor, Department of Surgery & Pediatrics, Children's Hospital at McMaster University Medical Centre, Hamilton, Ontario, Canada

Contents

CHAPTER 1

Introduction: radiological investigation of the neonate

John Mernagh
Haresh Kirpalani
Gerald Gill

THE TEAM APPROACH

The clinical examination and the radiological investigation together form the basis for the investigation of the acutely ill neonate. The proper use and interpretation of radiology requires good teamwork and communication between the clinician (including the perinatal obstetricians, and paediatric surgeons and neurosurgeons as appropriate) and the radiologist. In comparison with the adult patient there are specific concerns in the investigation of the neonate. In particular, the fragile nature of the neonate requires careful consideration of the risks and benefits of the investigations before they are performed. To facilitate this coordinated approach, regular rounds between the radiologists responsible for reporting the neonatal films and the clinical team are advised. Some hospitals choose to have daily work rounds between the clinical staff and the radiologists.

ROLE OF DIFFERENT IMAGE MODALITIES

Plain film radiography, ultrasonography (US), computed tomography, fluoroscopy and magnetic resonance imaging (MRI) all have important roles in the investigation of neonates. Nuclear medicine is used much less in these babies. All of these tests have specific uses and limitations, knowledge of which is necessary for their proper use.

Radiography and fluoroscopy

Before the advent of US and MRI, plain film radiography was the only method for the radiological investigation of the neonate. It still plays an important part. Principal concerns regarding the use of ionizing radiation (X-rays) relate to the critically ill neonate expected to undergo repeated examinations, sometimes over the course of years. Typically the radiation dose from a single chest/abdomen film would be 0.1 mSv (10 mrem) although this can vary widely with different techniques and equipment. A frequently overlooked precaution is gonadal shielding, important for future fertility. Estimates for the risk from radiation suggest an increase of one induced cancer over the lifetime of the patient for every 100 Sv (10 000 rem) radiation. Exposure in utero has been linked to childhood leukaemias (Mole 1990). The use of contrast poses a higher risk because of its allergic and nephrotoxic problems. If the film or image is approached by the clinician with the two questions below, it may be possible to minimize further radiation. These two questions are firstly a targeted question, and secondly an opportunistic question:

1. I have ordered this film for a specific reason – does the film allow me to address that reason?
2. Does the film show me any other possibly relevant information?

Proper technique is needed to ensure that follow-up examinations are compared adequately with previous examinations. This is particularly true of chest films, often done on portable machines.

Radiography and *computed tomography* are required in the investigation of the following:

1. Plain films for chest, abdomen and skeletal conditions. The chest X-ray (CXR) is still the test of choice in the investigation and follow-up of lung disease and bone disease. In the abdomen an X-ray is useful in assessing gas pattern in the bowel.
2. Computed tomography (CT) is useful in follow-up investigation of intracranial trauma, hypoxia and haemorrhage. More detailed examination of the head requires MRI. Generally CT is not useful in examination of the chest or abdomen of the neonate, although in rare instances of space-occupying lesions it may add some insight. CT allows one to measure density of tissues in Hounsfield units with water density at the zero point. Then fat and gas densities are in the minus range, soft tissue density ranges 20–150 and bone density 300+ units. This measurement allows one to distinguish between various tissues and also, by adding contrast intravenously and repeating the measurement, can distinguish between vascular and non-vascular structures.
3. Vascular and cardiac fluoroscopy including angiography. Fluoroscopy used with

contrast agents is useful for investigation of the gastrointestinal tract. Angiography is needed for specific problems usually related to thrombosis, but it should not be considered as a first-line investigation owing to its invasiveness, and again US has become the first choice.

Ultrasound

Ultrasonography is a rapidly expanding field which continues to play a key role in the investigation of the neonate, and moreover one that is finding increased applications. It does not require the use of ionizing radiation and thus eliminates any risks of X-rays. Doppler US is also important in assessing vascular patency and associated problems such as thrombosis. The portability of US equipment is also important as it allows for the bedside examination of even the critically ill neonate.

Ultrasound scans should be the first investigation in the following problems:

1. Intracranial haemorrhage. Ultrasonography is excellent in detecting and following subependymal, intraventricular and intraparenchymal haemorrhage. It is not reliable in detecting oedema or for examining the brain stem or posterior fossa. The US examination is limited by the size of the fontanelle as the ultrasound waves cannot penetrate bone. It is, however, readily repeatable. Further scans using CT or MRI may be necessary to clarify findings after the US examination.
2. Intracranial thrombosis. Doppler examination is the first study of choice in the investigation of superior sagittal or transverse sinus thrombosis in the neonate. In equivocal cases CT or MRI may be needed to verify the findings. Previously angiography would have been needed.
3. Abdomen and pelvis. Ultrasonography with or without Doppler is the first examination of choice in investigating the abdomen and pelvis. It allows for good visualization of abdominal and pelvic anatomy. It is of limited use for the detailed examination of the gastrointestinal tract for which contrast examinations are needed. Its primary limitation is that ultrasound waves cannot penetrate bowel gas. It has become the examination of choice in the investigation of pyloric stenosis.
4. Spine. As the neonatal spine is not fully calcified US is an excellent first examination for the spinal cord, particularly in the investigation of tethered cord. For detailed investigation MRI is needed.
5. Examination in utero. An ultrasound scan can be considered as a routine part of the intrauterine examination and can diagnose many neonatal problems before birth.

Magnetic resonance imaging

Magnetic resonance imaging provides superb anatomical delineation of structures, and is needed for the detailed investigation of the neonatal head and spine. It is not a first-line investigation, but is used to clarify findings of US or CT. Its greatest indication is in the area of congenital disorders such as the developmental disorders that are classified as gyral diseases and so-called neuronal cell migration defects. Its limitations are its availability, the need for anaesthesia in the neonate and the difficulty in monitoring.

Magnetic resonance imaging is the examination of choice in the investigation of intracranial pathology including congenital anomalies, trauma, hypoxic events and brain stem pathology.

Nuclear imaging

Nuclear imaging has limited use in the neonatal patient, primarily because of the advances made in ultrasound imaging in the past few years. It is still used for certain problems such as differentiating biliary atresia from neonatal hepatitis.

References

Mole R H 1990 Childhood cancer after prenatal exposure to diagnostic XR examination in Britain. British Journal of Cancer July 62(1): 152–168

CHAPTER 2

The chest

Haresh Kirpalani

John Mernagh

Mark Walton

Pamela Cairns

Gerald Gill

INDICATIONS FOR CHEST X-RAY

The plain film of the chest remains the single most frequently requested test in neonatology. It is used primarily to assess the state of the lungs, the size and shape of the heart, the position of an endotracheal tube (ETT), chest drains, nasogastric tubes and vascular lines. Although the chest X-ray (CXR) may be used as an initial screen for several disease processes it is often followed by more specific investigations – for instance, if congenital heart disease is suspected, by echocardiography.

TECHNICAL CONSIDERATIONS

The CXR requires a surprisingly high degree of skill to obtain consistently good images in the neonatal intensive care unit as the technician has to consider:

1. minimal exposure factors (low kV and mAs)
2. patient motion (squirming)
3. respiratory motion (ventilator rate)
4. the constraints of working within a confined space upon a premature infant with multiple lines and tubes.

Common technical problems

1. Films in expiration may be misinterpreted as showing a worsening in the clinical condition (Fig. 2.1).
2. Rotated films: one lung may be partially obscured and appear smaller. Figure 2.2a is normal and shows symmetry, while Figure 2.2b is rotated and shows asymmetry of the ribs and clavicles.
3. Lordotic films: the cardiac apex appears elevated as in right ventricular hypertrophy. Lordosis also influences the appearance of the level at which the ETT is lying (Fig. 2.3).
4. Comparing technically light and dark films (i.e. the penetration) in a sequence may lead to errors of misinterpretation. To assess penetration, look for the density of the spine and soft tissues (Fig. 2.4a). In the 'overpenetrated' film, for instance, the arms 'appear to disappear' (Fig. 2.4b). In addition, the umbilical venous line is placed too high.

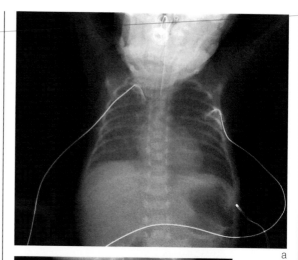

a

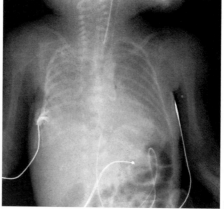

b

Fig. 2.1 Chest X-ray: (a) inspiratory; (b) expiratory. The expiratory film may be misinterpreted as a worsening in clinical condition.

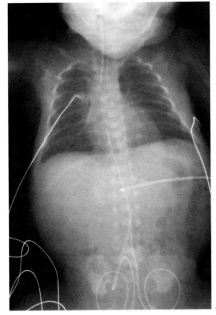

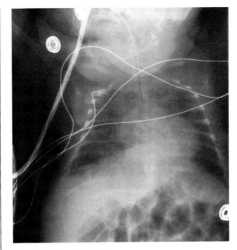

Fig. 2.3 Lordotic film.

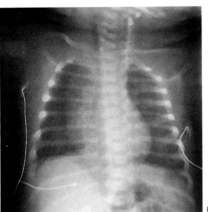

Fig. 2.2 Chest X-ray: (a) normal film; (b) rotated film.

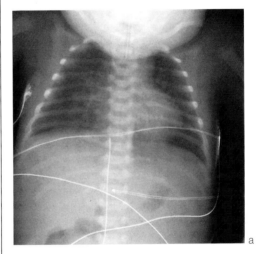

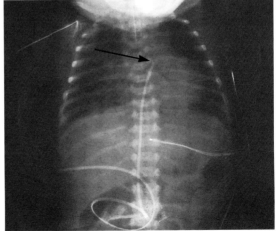

Fig. 2.4 Comparison of 'light' (a) and 'dark' (b) films. Note high right venous line in (b) (arrow).

THE 'NORMAL' NEONATAL CHEST X-RAY

The heart and thymus are prominent features but over 24 hours of postnatal life the thymus usually 'involutes', especially with stress. Figure 2.5a shows a baby with minimal interstitial markings and a large mediastinum; on follow-up, Figure 2.5b, this has involuted. Often in infants weighing less than 750 g the thymus appears much smaller, and it may not be seen even on the initial CXR (Fig. 2.5c).

Interpreting the heart size is difficult when there is rotation, or varying degrees of expiration and various amounts of positive pressure ventilation. A cardiothoracic ratio therefore requires good films. A normal upper limit is often cited is a cardiothoracic ratio of less than 65%. Pulmonary vessels are usually indistinct (see Chapter 3).

Pulmonary fissures are seen infrequently. If seen, an underlying pathophysiological condition may be present, e.g. retained lung fluid in transient tachypnoea of the newborn (TTN). Since the fissures are not well seen, the lung lobes are often not well defined in the neonatal lung. We therefore often refer to the lung 'zones' rather than lung 'lobes'; but admittedly, this nomenclature is not universal. Major bronchi may be seen in the perihilar area, especially through the heart, as for example in Figure 2.5a. This is a normal finding, and should not be confused with the peripheral air bronchogram of hyaline membrane disease (HMD).

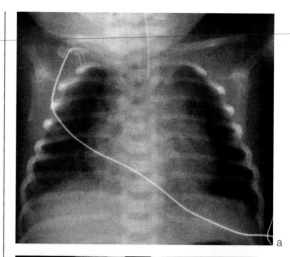

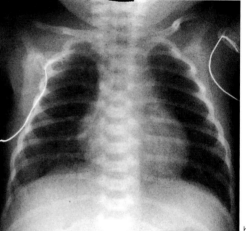

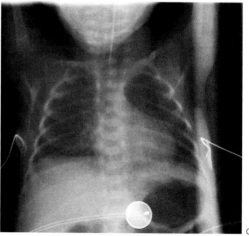

Fig. 2.5 Normal CXR. A prominent thymus (a) usually involutes over 24 hours (b); in infants < 750 g it may not be visible at all (c).

THE ABNORMAL CHEST X-RAY

A density in the CXR is non-specific, and represents replacement of the normal airway and alveoli with abnormal material. From the CXR alone aspirated fluid, pulmonary haemorrhage, pulmonary infection and some forms of cardiac failure cannot be distinguished. For example, the 'white-out' pattern of severe hyaline membrane disease often seen on the initial film is radiologically indistinguishable from the CXR 'white-out' pattern of severe pulmonary haemorrhage in an infant who has deteriorated, with bloody fluid coming up the endotracheal tube, and who may have clinical signs of a patent ductus arteriosus (PDA). The correct interpretation of a CXR 'white-out' depends upon the timing of the clinical features.

Scoring systems

There are several scoring systems to gauge severity of lung disease in newborns. These include scores for acute disease such as HMD (Tudor et al 1976) and for the changes of bronchopulmonary dysplasia such as those of Weinstein et al (1995). These formal scoring systems are not widely used except in research protocols, but the beginner may find that they provide some structure initially, to be superseded by clinical experience.

Using the CXR as a guide to lung volume and cardiac filling

Clinical measurement of lung volumes is difficult, but CXRs may provide clinically relevant information. In the future computer-assisted lung volume derivation from CXR images may be helpful (Kirpalani et al 1997). Currently, clinical observation of respiratory excursions, coupled with inspection of the CXR for the degree of lung filling as reflected by diaphragmatic depth, is the best approach. Diaphragmatic depth is thought to be good if 8–10 ribs are seen above the diaphragm.

The sequence in Figures 2.6–2.9 illustrates the difficulty in the clinical trade-off between lung recruitment and overdistension. The example illustrated is an infant with chronic lung disease of 32 weeks gestational age at birth, at a chronological age of 36 weeks. Collapse of the right lung precipitated severe hypoxaemia and hypercarbia and cardiovascular collapse (Fig. 2.6). Switching to high-frequency oscillation (HFO) resulted in clinical improvement, but HFO at a high mean airway pressure restricted filling volume as seen in the decreased heart size (Fig. 2.7). Furthermore, the 'better' lung became hyperinflated and emphysematous with mediastinal shift (Fig. 2.8); and then ruptured with an air leak (Fig. 2.9). The infant survived with no clinical or major radiological sequelae. These conditions are discussed further below.

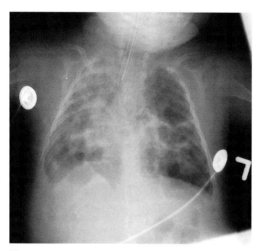

Fig. 2.6

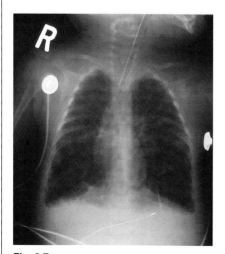

Fig. 2.7

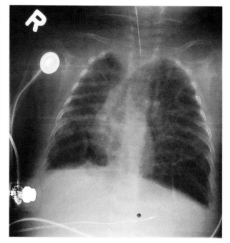

Fig. 2.8

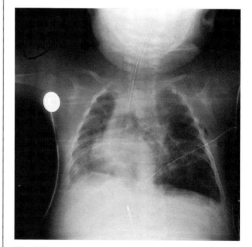

Fig. 2.9

RESPIRATORY DISTRESS SYNDROME AND HYALINE MEMBRANE DISEASE

Clinical signs of respiratory distress are expiratory grunting, use of accessory muscles, indrawing, and tachypnoea (> 60 breaths per minute) with cyanosis, implying hypoxia and hypercapnia. The infant may require varying degrees of respiratory support including oxygen, continuous positive airway pressure (CPAP) and intermittent positive pressure ventilation (IPPV). The clinical signs are non-specific. A correct diagnosis depends primarily on the clinical history, but the CXR appearance may help rule out some conditions. The CXR is also required to check for ETT positions, presence of air leaks, lung volume recruitment and response to therapy, and to consider cardiac disorders.

There are many causes of respiratory distress syndrome (RDS). Hyaline membrane disease is one cause of RDS, secondary to surfactant deficiency. This is considered to be primary in prematurity (less than 37 weeks gestational age). Surfactant deficiency may also occur following disorders such as asphyxia, meconium aspiration, maternal diabetes, or infection, in which case it is a secondary RDS. The X-ray appearances are indistinguishable. Both primary and secondary RDS may benefit from therapy with exogenous surfactant.

Radiological appearance

There are three characteristic radiographic features of HMD:

1. low-volume lungs
2. air bronchograms
3. fine, granular lung pattern.

These features are progressive but may be altered by ventilation strategy or surfactant therapy. Mild disease is seen as a diffuse, linear granular pattern which is usually uniform. The term 'ground glass' is often used to describe the appearance of this and moderate disease (Fig. 2.10). Moderate disease shows the appearance of peripheral air bronchograms (i.e. **not** behind the cardiac shadow), with the cardiac border blurred (Fig. 2.11). In severe disease the lung fields are

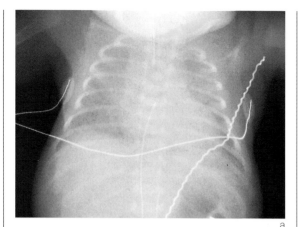

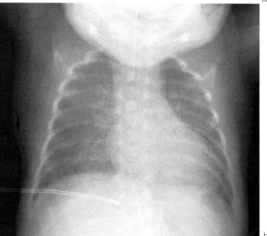

Fig. 2.10 Two films in an infant with RDS taken 1 day apart. Note the typical 'ground glass' appearance in the first image (a). The second image (b) is taken after surfactant therapy, showing marked clearing of lung water or better recruitment of lung segments.

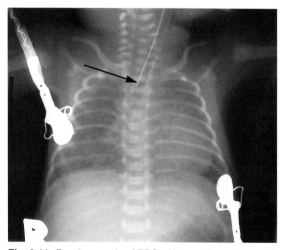

Fig. 2.11 Good example of RDS with granular pattern and air bronchograms. ETT in good position (arrow).

completely opaque and indistinguishable from the cardiac shadow (white-out).

Lung volume is not a very specific sign and may be altered with positive pressure ventilation, as described above.

An example of incorrect ETT placement is shown in Figure 2.12.

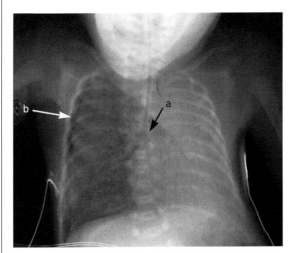

Fig. 2.12 Example of endotracheal tube placed with its distal tip in the right main bronchus, aerating the right lung only (arrow a). Note small right pneumothorax (arrow b), left lung totally collapsed.

Secondary RDS

Especially in infants of more than 37 weeks gestational age, consider other causes of RDS than prematurity. These are where initial surfactant sufficiency becomes inadequate, resulting in a 'secondary' surfactant deficiency.

- Hypoxia or shock and underperfusion from any cause will exacerbate surfactant deficiency.
- Infections are clinically and radiologically often impossible to distinguish from RDS. Treatment usually includes antibiotics for 48 hours until culture is negative. Radiography may reveal areas of consolidation and/or streakiness (Fig. 2.13).
- Aspiration syndrome is discussed below (Fig. 2.14).
- Infants of diabetic mothers may have RDS and also cardiac enlargement (Fig. 2.15). The latter results from hypoglycaemia, and may be associated with hypertrophic obstructive cardiomyopathy, visible by two-dimensional echocardiography. It resolves spontaneously. Some infants appear to have 'immature' surfactant.

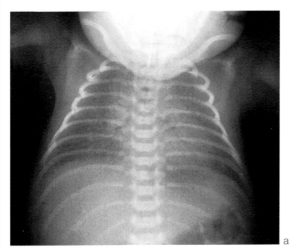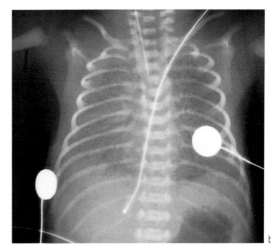

a   b

Fig. 2.13 Two different patients (a,b) with beta-haemolytic streptococcal infection.

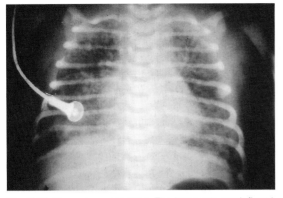

Fig. 2.14 Meconium aspiration. The lungs are overinflated (out pouching between ribs) and there are patchy areas of coarse increased density. Infections, particularly GBS, may have a similar pattern.

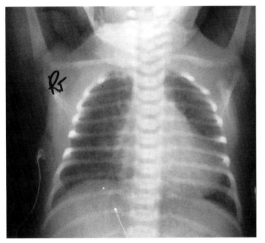

Fig. 2.15 Infant of a diabetic mother showing cardiomegaly.

TRANSIENT TACHYPNOEA OF THE NEWBORN

Transient tachypnoea of the newborn (TTN) is a delay in the normal transition of the fetal lung to extrauterine life. It is commonly seen in those born by caesarean section to a non-labouring mother, but can also occur following vaginal delivery. This delay prevents the normal catecholamine-induced reversal in the lung of fluid efflux to fluid absorption, which normally takes place in the course of labour.

Clinical features

The majority of infants have minimal to moderate respiratory distress with only modest requirements for therapy. Two complications may be seen. If infants are allowed to become hypoxic they may develop persistent pulmonary hypertension; some infants may develop a secondary surfactant deficiency. The process is self-limited in the majority of infants, who establish absorption of lung fluid within 48 hours following birth.

Radiological appearance

The CXR typically shows mildly overexpanded, hazy lungs, with prominent fissures and occasionally pleural effusions. Group B streptococcal or other infections or aspiration cannot confidently be radiologically differentiated. Figure 2.16 shows two films taken 1 day apart of a neonate with TTN.

IMMATURE LUNG SYNDROME

Immature lung syndrome (ILS) is often seen in infants with a birthweight below 750 g, an initially clear lung on CXR, and minimal oxygen requirements. A microatelectasis with diffuse densities develops, associated with an increasing oxygen requirement and (by the end of the first week of life) increased ventilatory requirements. This is partly due to the very compliant chest wall of these infants, and partly to diaphragmatic fatigue and associated apnoea. Loss of lung volume leads to scarring and an appearance almost indistinguishable from bronchopulmonary dysplasia (BPD). This condition was first termed 'chronic pulmonary insufficiency of prematurity' (CPIP) by Krauss et al (1975) and has prompted a new definition of BPD (see below).

The baby shown in Figures 2.17–2.20 had 32 CXRs over a 6-week period, of which four are shown here.

AIR LEAK SYNDROMES

Air leak syndromes result from lung rupture, often associated with IPPV. All such syndromes are considered as 'baro-volu-trauma' to the lung, and may progress to chronic lung disease or BPD.

Clinical features

'Spontaneous' pneumothorax can be associated with the first breath, or with resuscitation. Occasional renal anomalies are associated. In the delivery room pneumothorax is one possible cause of a failure to resuscitate the newborn. Consider emergency drainage in this context if everything appropriate has been done. (Is the endotracheal tube in the right place? Is the

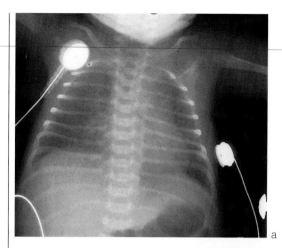

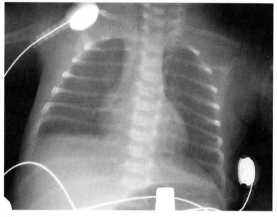

Fig. 2.16 (a) Granularity is seen in both lungs, with a differential diagnosis of RDS, TTN, infection and patent ductus arteriosus. Here the appearance is more 'hazy' than 'granular' and the fissure is a contributory feature to the X-ray diagnosis. Notice the indistinctness of the lower left lung abutting onto the heart. (b) One day later, without any specific treatment, there has been clearing of the granular appearance of both lungs.

infant receiving chest compressions correctly? etc.) Air leaks later may complicate RDS, aspiration syndromes and/or IPPV. Outside the delivery room, there may be a sudden worsened respiratory distress plus decreased movement, or a sudden increase in ventilation requirements. Decreased air entry on the affected side may be difficult to detect in very small infants. If large air leaks are present, cardiovascular collapse may be profound, requiring volume and inotropic support. This

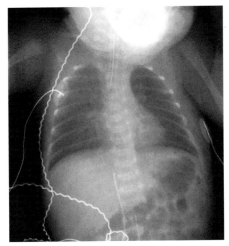

Fig. 2.17 Immature lung syndrome. In the first hours of postnatal life, a clear CXR with a normal appearance is seen, with no significant air bronchograms, although the child is intubated.

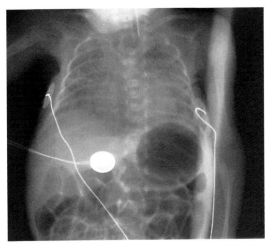

Fig. 2.19 By day 6 the lungs are poorly expanded with marked interstitial and alveolar densities.

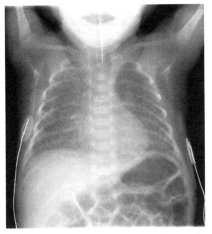

Fig. 2.18 On day 4 the lungs are less well expanded and an interstitial pattern is developing.

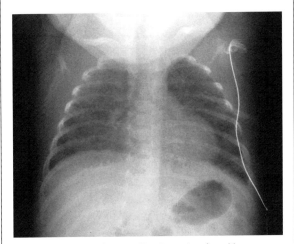

Fig. 2.20 Finally, after needing 6 weeks of positive pressure ventilation and oxygen requirements, the infant is extubated; the CXR shows near-normality, although some residual interstitial density is apparent.

cardiovascular system collapse implies mediastinal shift (tension pneumothorax). In dramatic deteriorations, a 'blind' needle aspiration, sometimes preceded by illumination of the chest for a large leak, is advisable without awaiting a CXR. In the delivery room context this is especially so. If small, pneumothoraces may not need drainage unless the infant has to be transported.

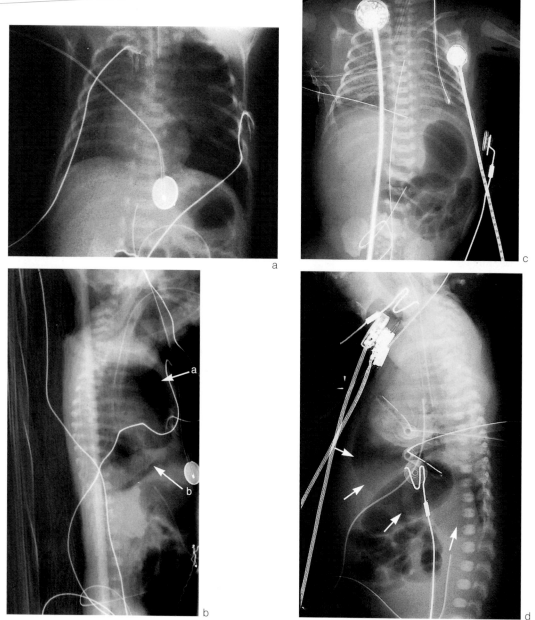

Fig. 2.21 Pneumothorax. Anteroposterior (a) and lateral (b) views of the chest with a 'clear' cardiac border on the AP film. The lateral film shows that the 'clarity' is actually an increased lucency due to free air, on the left side. Note that arrow a by itself may indicate only a pneumomediastinum; but arrow b indicates a pneumothorax with free air outlining the diaphragm. Another patient (c, d) shows two right-sided chest tubes in place treating a pneumothorax; (d) shows the lateral view, in which the lower tube is seen to turn posteriorly under the right lung into a good position, where there is a large pocket of air (multiple arrows). The second and higher chest tube, however, is likely to be penetrating the lung. Especially in this circumstance ensure that the tube is truly bubbling. If not, consider its withdrawal and replacement.

Radiological appearance

As infants are lying flat, the free air is anterior to the lung and therefore an edge of collapsed lung may not be visible. In reading a CXR for potential air leaks the lateral film can be helpful where there is a 'clear' cardiac border on the anteroposterior (AP) film. The lateral film may show that the 'clarity' is actually an increased lucency due to free air (Fig. 2.21). In addition the lateral film is useful for correct placement of chest tubes and ensuring that free air has been released (Fig. 2.21). Check that the tip of the tube lies within the air pocket to be drained, that the perforations on the catheter are within the pleural space, and finally that the tip of the tube is not past the midline. The lateral film may also help to define the position of draining chest tubes and may assist in avoiding 'shish-kebab' lungs or lung perforation. Other examples of pneumothorax are illustrated in Figures 2.22–2.26.

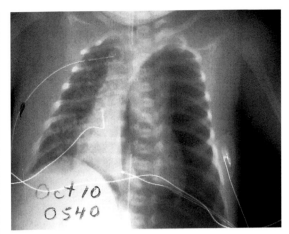

Fig. 2.23 The same infant as in the previous figure, 2 days later. The right air leak is drained, and there is now a large left tension pneumothorax with deviation of midline structures and inferior displacement of the left hemidiaphragm.

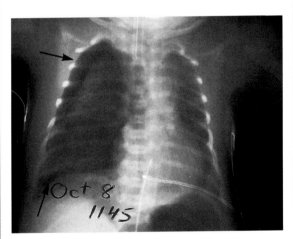

Fig. 2.22 Right-sided pneumothorax showing lucency between right lateral chest wall and lung, also see rim above diaphragm (arrows). Note that 'stiff lungs' do not collapse easily.

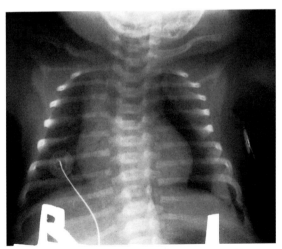

Fig. 2.24 Moderate-sized medial pneumothorax. Air collecting medial to the lung as seen here can be confused with a pneumopericardium. A right clavicular fracture is also seen. Examine for position of pneumomediastinum. Suspect this when the thymic shadow is separated from the heart.

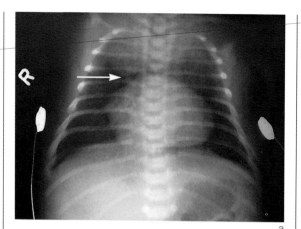

a

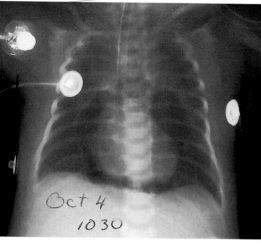

Fig. 2.26 Anteroposterior film of another patient with pneumomediastinum. There is a faint lucency overlying the mid-thorax. The thymus is seen outlining the superior lateral aspects; this is easily confused with a pneumopericardium. But if compared to Figure 2.27, Figure 2.26 lacks a confining boundary of the pericardial sac – so-called 'tram line' sign. Even so, it may only be resolved by either a lateral view and/or an echo.

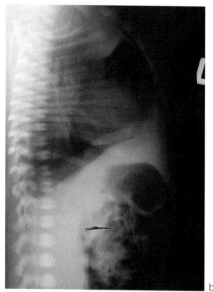

b

Fig. 2.25 Anteroposterior (a) and lateral (b) films showing elevation of thymus by mediastinal air. Note 'sail' sign of thymus on the AP film (arrow).

Other sites of extrapulmonary air include:

- Pneumopericardium (Fig. 2.27).
- Pneumoperitoneum – this may be a manifestation of pulmonary air leak or bowel perforation (Fig. 2.28).
- Disseminated intravascular air embolism – this is rare; it is almost always fatal (Fig. 2.29).
- Pulmonary interstitial emphysema – see below.

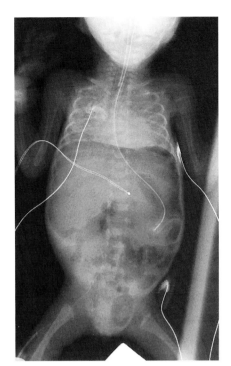

Fig. 2.28 Pneumoperitoneum with a large amount of free air below the diaphragm outlining liver, spleen and bowel loops. Incidentally, note the left inguinal hernia.

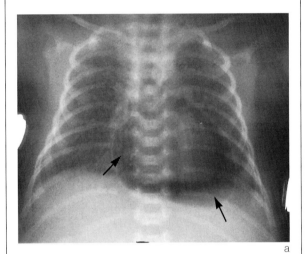

a

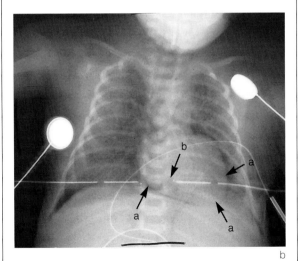

b

Fig. 2.27 Pneumopericardium. A thin line of pericardium can be seen just lateral to pericardial air (arrows labelled a); this was then drained. Note the cardiac silhouette tamponaded first in (a) and released later in (b). The tip of the drain is within the pericardium (arrow b).

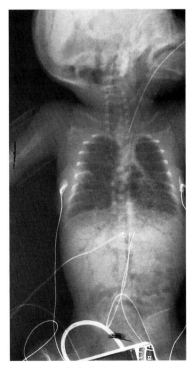

Fig. 2.29 Gross interstitial air plus vascular air in cardiac silhouette and in major arterial vessels. Note also air in the cerebral sagittal sinus and cerebral ventricles.

Pulmonary interstitial emphysema

Pulmonary interstitial emphysema (PIE) is alveolar rupture into the peribronchial spaces, tracking along the lymphatic channels, leading to an air accumulation within the pulmonary interstitium. Often, it follows high-pressure ventilation, with deteriorating oxygenation. The general treatment is to minimize further 'baro-volu-trauma'. Some advocate the use of steroids. On chest X-ray, PIE may be diffuse or localized (Figs 2.30–2.35). Irregular air densities (dark areas) appear in the interstitium of the lung, often with a vague orientation towards the hilum. This condition can be mistaken for improvement in HMD, as the lungs often look better-expanded and darker. In areas of dramatic local hyperinflation (most commonly the left lower lobe), local treatment can be attempted if one side can be occluded (e.g. by selective intubation or balloon inflation).

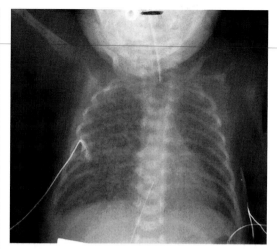

Fig. 2.30 Generalized PIE: coarse, irregular air densities throughout the lung fields, with a bubbly appearance, oriented towards the hilum. The air density is unlike the 'finer' air bronchogram and granularity of HMD.

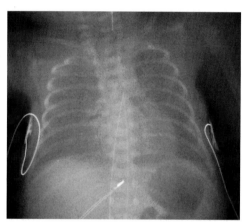

Fig. 2.31 Day 1 of life, showing HMD with diffuse granular pattern and air bronchograms. The evolution of PIE can be seen in Figures 2.32–2.35.

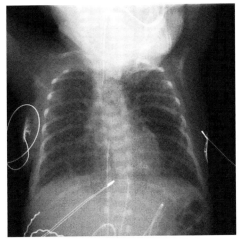

Fig. 2.32 Day 2 of life, showing PIE bilaterally, more prominent on the left.

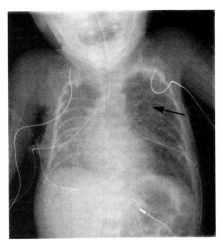

Fig. 2.34 Day 13 of life, showing poor expansion of right lobe and overexpansion of left lobe. Note a 2 cm cyst above the left hilum (arrow).

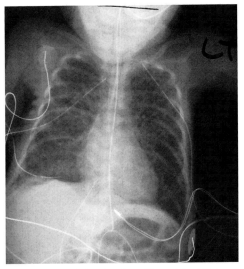

Fig. 2.33 Day 11 of life, showing diffuse interstitial pattern. Small cystic changes are seen bilaterally. Two chest tubes have been placed to drain pneumothoraces.

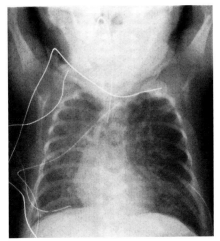

Fig. 2.35 Day 15 of life, showing overexpansion of the left lobe displacing the upper mediastinum to right. Note several small cysts in the left lung peripherally.

Iatrogenic PIE and its problems The sequence of films in Figures 2.36–2.42 is an instructive series, as it shows how attention to small detail is vital and if ignored may lead to serious sequelae for very low birthweight infants. It shows an early misplaced tube with air leak; then local PIE; then the onset of severe collapse of the lung on that side; then a persistent difficulty in recruiting lung volume with onset of BPD and severe lung disease with PDA; and finally, improvement with steroids. We conclude that because the low position of the ETT in the first hours of life was unrecognized, the tube was not withdrawn, which led to further damage of the right lung. Despite appropriate management of the pneumothorax and PIE, this markedly prolonged the clinical course.

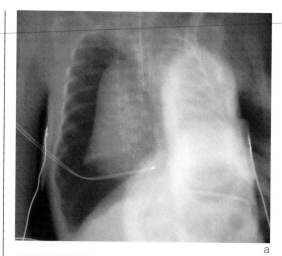

a

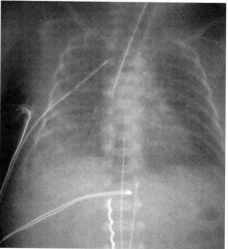

b

Fig. 2.36 Iatrogenic PIE: the first hours of life. (a) The ETT in the right main bronchus causing a right tension pneumothorax and collapse of the left lung. (b) The pneumothorax has been drained by a chest tube, but the ETT remains low. It is however aerating the left lung. The right lower zones are not completely expanded.

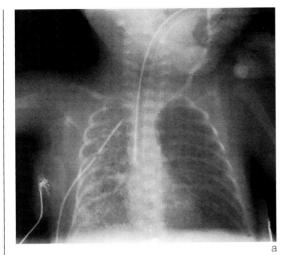

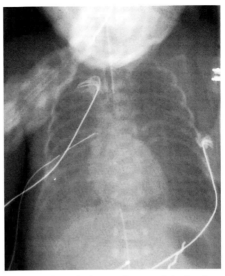

Fig. 2.38 Despite increasing ventilator treatment, only part of the right lung has been recruited. The right lower zones, the area of previous PIE, appear dense.

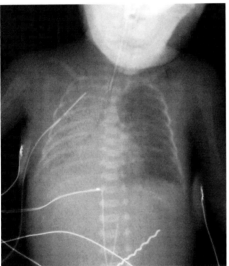

Fig. 2.37 Day 2 of life. (a) With the ETT still in a low position, PIE is developing in the right lung, especially in the right lower zones. (b) By 28 hours of age, there is collapse of the right lung even though the ETT has been withdrawn to a satisfactory position. We conjecture that the trauma to the right lung has already been caused, leading to the subsequent prolonged course with BPD and treatment.

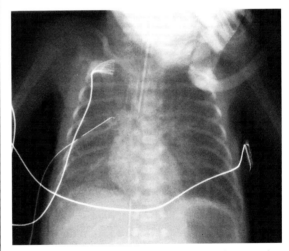

Fig. 2.39 By 1 week of age there is still some increased density in the right lower zone, with a fine interstitial pattern of early chronic lung disease.

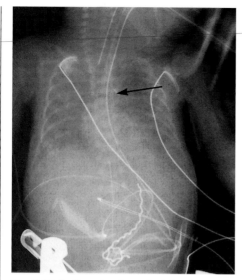

Fig. 2.40 By 2 weeks of age the infant has undergone a duct ligation (note clip and arrow). Despite this he has considerable bilateral densities, probably the early changes of BPD.

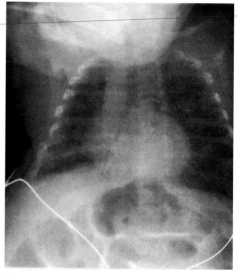

Fig. 2.42 By 14 weeks of age, the infant is on low-flow oxygen and still on steroids, and CXR still shows the hyperexpansion of BPD.

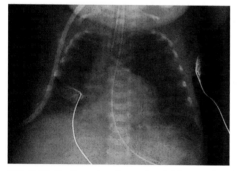

Fig. 2.41 By 8 weeks of age steroid therapy has improved the densities; however, the typical hyperexpansion and coarse interstitial pattern of later BPD are evident.

NECROTIZING TRACHEOBRONCHITIS

A special form of air leak can present with a tracheal block syndrome associated with severe baro-volu-trauma. The classic triad is a rising and profound hypercarbia with an inability to move the chest despite very high ventilatory pressures, and severe air leaks. Rigid bronchoscopy with removal of necrotic airway tissue and mucus hypersecretions can be life-saving, as can saline instillation, immediately followed by vigorous hand-bagging and suction. Figure 2.43 shows an infant who following meconium aspiration developed severe persistent pulmonary hypertension. This was treated with hyperventilation, and resulted in baro-volu-trauma.

Bronchography is rarely done; a film showing the sequelae of severe necrotizing bronchitis is shown in Figure 2.44.

BRONCHOPULMONARY DYSPLASIA

Bronchopulmonary dysplasia (BPD) was originally recognized by radiologists, who noted that infants who previously had died of respiratory failure were now surviving but with a chronic respiratory insufficiency associated with radiological scarring (Northway et al 1974). Baro-volu-trauma and oxygen toxicity produce an early acute inflammatory lung response which subsides into chronic inflammation. This is accompanied by a usually slow but nevertheless inexorable fibrosis, which results in areas of hyperinflation and areas of collapse. There are nowadays two commonly used clinical definitions. An older definition stated that BPD was the diagnosis in a preterm infant who had RDS, was ventilated, and at 28 days of age still had an FiO_2 greater than 30% and an abnormal CXR (Bancalari et al 1979). A later definition was thought necessary, as it was noted that the majority of extremely premature infants (< 28 weeks gestational age) fulfilled the above definition. The increased survival rate makes an increased oxygen requirement at over 37 weeks corrected age more appropriate (Shennan et al 1988); see immature lung syndrome, above.

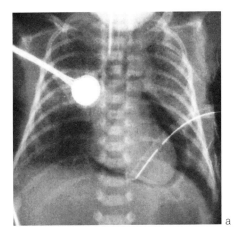

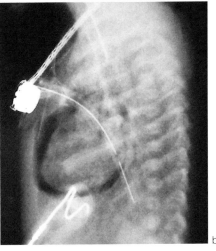

Fig. 2.43 Dramatic presentation of baro-volu-trauma with a pneumopericardium, seen in posteroanterior (a) and lateral (b) views with a drain.

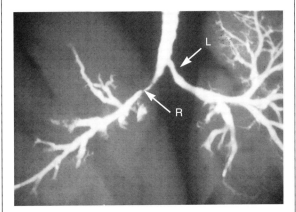

Fig. 2.44 Bronchogram showing the sequela of severe necrotizing bronchitis, with stricture in the right and left mainstem bronchus (arrows).

Clinical features

Prolonged oxygen and/or need for mechanical ventilation, associated with an abnormal CXR, are the hallmarks of BPD. The infant has ventilation-perfusion mismatch, increased airway reactivity, and in severe cases cor pulmonale. Steroid treatment helps considerably but carries complications such as hypertension, glycosuria, cardiomyopathy, growth failure and osteoporosis; most recently concerns have been raised about adverse long-term neurodevelopmental effects.

Radiological appearance

The disease is characterized by coarse interstitial densities, interspersed with cyst-like areas, which progress to general hyperinflation with larger cysts. In later stages linear densities develop in the lungs. Correspondingly, right ventricular strain may show with enlargement suggestive of cor pulmonale. These series of changes may occur over weeks to months. Figures 2.45–2.51 show this series of events in one baby, starting with a small, immature lung. Partly due to both antenatal and prenatal steroids, this type of severe outcome is less commonly seen at present.

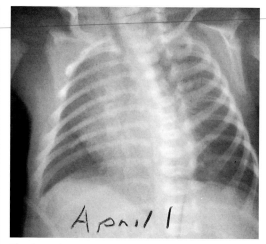

Fig. 2.45 Bronchopulmonary dysplasia. Day 1 of life, shows a rotated film; however, the lungs are clear. The appearances are those of 'immature lung syndrome' not HMD/RDS.

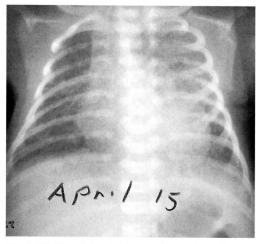

Fig. 2.46 Film at day 15 shows microatelectasis, decreased lung volume and some increased densities, with some cardiomegaly.

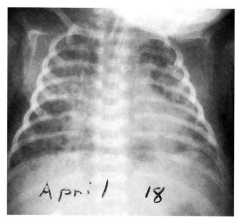

Fig. 2.47 Film from day 18 shows a coarse interstitial pattern with small cystic areas.

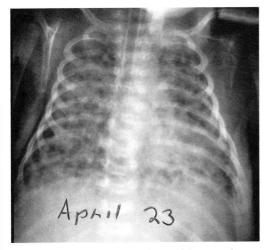

Fig. 2.48 Day 23: the coarse interstitial pattern is more obvious, and there are increased cystic changes.

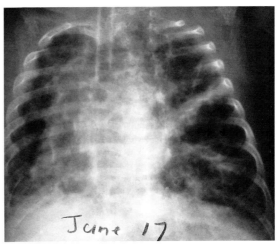

Fig. 2.50 Film from day 70 shows the marked bullae which distort the entire lung parenchyma. Overinflation is increased.

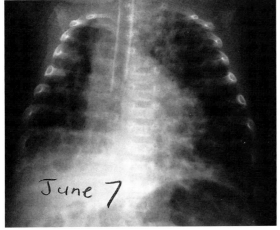

Fig. 2.49 By day 60, the infant has developed marked overinflation with a barrel-shaped chest. The coarse interstitial densities are finer, almost linear. The ETT is too far down. Note the 'lifting' of the heart apex from the diaphragm, showing right ventriculomegaly.

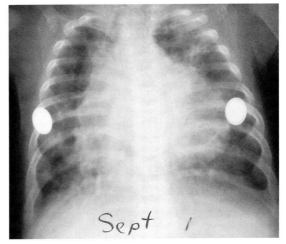

Fig. 2.51 Film from day 148 showing fully developed cor pulmonale with marked cardiomegaly. Note the lungs are clearer, suggestive of pulmonary hypertension with oligaemic lungs.

The sequence of films in Figures 2.52–2.57 demonstrates a chronic respiratory insufficiency indistinguishable from BPD. This resulted from a multifactorial process comprising an initial ventilator dependency and some pulmonary hypoplasia in an infant with a large omphalocele at birth. This infant later had severe gastrooesophageal reflux and repeated aspirations, and also several episodes of cardiac failure associated with steroid therapy from chronic ventilator dependency.

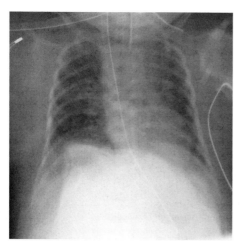

Fig. 2.52 This film shows the omphalocele (as soft tissue over the anterior abdomen) (see text) and small lungs with an interstitial pattern; these lesions are associated with pulmonary hypoplasia.

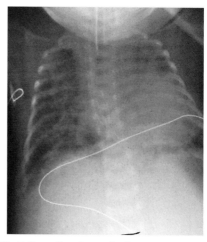

Fig. 2.54 At 2 months of age, the lungs are overexpanded with a chronic interstitial pattern, and cardiomegaly persists.

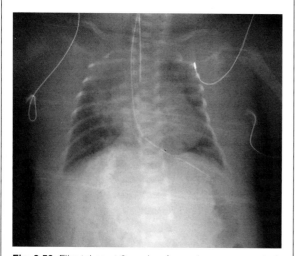

Fig. 2.53 Film taken at 2 weeks of age shows a corrected omphalocele, but there is cardiomegaly and pulmonary consolidation. Note the increased soft tissue swelling associated with the need for large-volume replacement therapy.

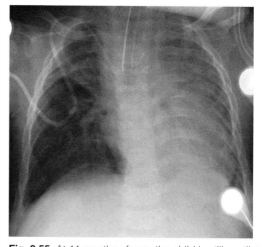

Fig. 2.55 At 11 months of age, the child is still ventilator-dependent with overexpanded lungs, and now has consolidation in the left lower lobe and partial right upper lobe atelectasis.

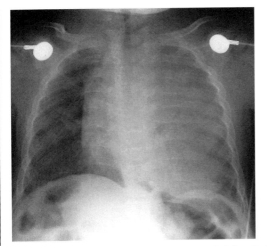

Fig. 2.56 At 18 months of age, there was a brief period where the child was able to be extubated; but the lungs remain overexpanded, and cardiomegaly persists.

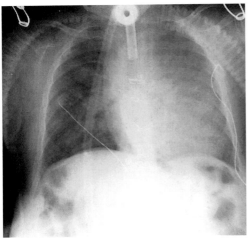

Fig. 2.57 At 22 months of age, the child is developing normally for speech and intelligence, but is ventilated at home via a tracheostomy, and has had a fundus wrap-around (fundoplication) to prevent severe reflux and aspirations. The wire sutures in the sternum are visible, as is the tubing of the home ventilator.

WILSON–MIKITY SYNDROME

Wilson–Mikity syndrome is a type of 'pure' oxygen toxicity resulting in chronic lung disease, which was more common before the advent of mechanical ventilation (Wilson & Mikity 1960). It is likely that the disease has altered its radiological manifestations as a result of positive pressure baro-volu-trauma, resulting in a picture of broncho-pulmonary dysplasia.

Radiological appearance

The radiological features are similar to BPD, with a coarse interstitial pattern and the development of cystic changes. A typical example is shown in Figure 2.58.

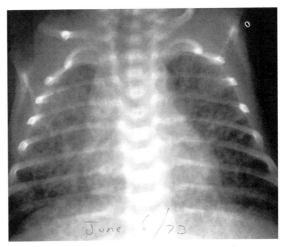

Fig. 2.58 An infant near term, with moderate RDS requiring respiratory support with ventilation and oxygen. A moderately coarse interstitial pattern has developed, similar in appearance to BPD but with a coarser, 'lacier' look to it, meaning cystic lucencies. These lesions may resolve at any of the stages, or may progress to chronic lung disease with hypertension and right heart failure – i.e. cor pulmonale.

PNEUMONIA

Pneumonias in the newborn often give rise to respiratory distress, and are a frequent cause of morbidity in newborns, though they are also often difficult to prove bacteriologically. Many infections present with non-specific features such as RDS, poor perfusion, jaundice or lethargy. Two presentations can be distinguished on the basis of time.

Early presentation

This is usually one of respiratory distress, with or without other clinical evidence of sepsis such as shock. This presentation is often indistinguishable from RDS due to 'pure' surfactant deficiency. The CXR pattern is often exactly the same. The differential diagnosis may be impossible to establish with certainty, although the following may help: the presence of amniotic fluid infection; prolonged rupture of membranes; amnionitis; and elevated band cell counts in infant blood.

Most authorities recommend treatment with antibiotics, stopped if within 48 hours there are negative cultures. Most early infections are with either group B streptococci or coliforms. Occasionally fungal infections or viral infections may present with unusual features; the latter especially may cause myocarditis with cardiac failure.

Late presentation

Late presentation with similar symptoms often occurs with nosocomial infections. The most common infective organism is coagulase-negative *Staphylococcus epidermidis*. *Candida* is also a likely organism, especially in very low-birthweight infants, who have had long lines in situ and perhaps repeated courses of antibiotics (see Chapter 6). Again, antibiotic treatment pending negative culture is advised.

Radiological appearance

Firm diagnosis is impossible from radiographic appearance alone, but compared with HMD, the lungs are more expanded and the densities are often more patchy. Localized lobar pneumonias are unusual in the newborn, and are most commonly due to a misplaced ETT or collapse with obstruction.

Specific infections

Group B streptococcal infection

Clinical features Women are commonly colonized with group B streptococci (GBS), although the frequency varies according to locality. The neonate can acquire infections in the prepartum, intrapartum or postpartum periods. There are two general forms of presentation: an early presentation at 1–5 days of life is usually a respiratory illness, whereas a late presentation at 5–28 days of life is usually meningitis. However, an overlap between the early and late forms is frequent.

The presentation is as for pneumonias in general. However, in addition features of persistent pulmonary hypertension of the newborn (PPHN) are frequent in this infection (see below). Overwhelming sepsis with GBS and PPHN is not easy to deal with and mortality is high.

Radiological appearance The CXR appearance can vary widely from a minimal widespread interstitial pattern to a dense homogeneous infiltrate (Figs 2.59–2.61).

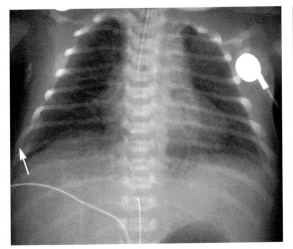

Fig. 2.59 Infection with GBS. A single film of the chest shows diffuse, increased, coarse interstitial markings. The granularity associated with this raises a differential diagnosis of RDS or HMD. Note the right-sided pleural effusion (arrow).

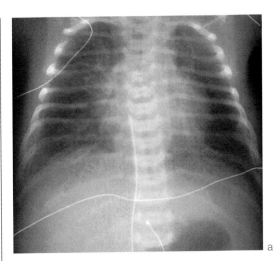

a

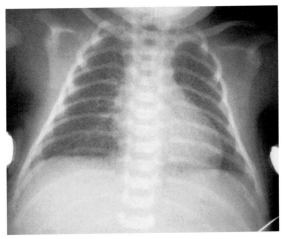

Fig. 2.60 A second example of GBS infection in a neonate, this time showing a fine granular pattern in the lungs. Again, the differential diagnosis is RDS or HMD. In this case the granularity is somewhat coarser than normal for HMD, and there is no significant air bronchogram.

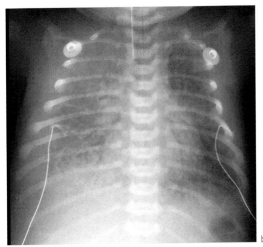

b

Fig. 2.61 Two cases of GBS pneumonia showing coarse interstitial markings. Both have right pleural effusions and smaller left pleural effusions (a, b). Note the range of severity of the interstitial markings; both interstitial and alveolar markings are much more severe in (b) than in (a).

Staphylococcal (aureus) pneumonia

Clinical features Staphylococcal infection is rare in neonates, but when it occurs it may lead to long-term complications with pneumatoceles as shown in Figures 2.62–2.65. The rare possibility of immune disorders needs to be ruled out in such situations.

Radiological appearance Staphylococcal pneumonias usually give rise to extensive air space consolidation, sometimes with pleural fluid, and occasionally pneumatoceles. Figures 2.62–2.65 are a series of films showing the development and resolution of severe staphylococcal pneumonia in a neonate.

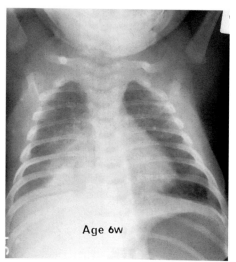

Fig. 2.62 Staphylococcal pneumonia. The first film of the sequence shows right middle and lower lobe parenchyma consolidation. Note that the right heart border cannot be seen, indicating right middle lobe involvement (silhouette sign). The left lung is clear. There is no pleural effusion on the right.

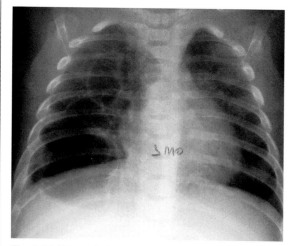

Fig. 2.64 Six weeks later there has been practically complete clearing of the consolidation within the right lung. There has been coalescence and enlargement of the pneumatoceles, particularly in the lower lobe region.

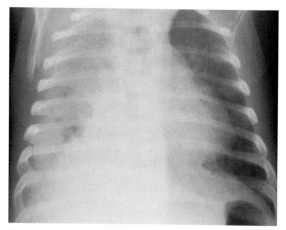

Fig. 2.63 Film taken 2 days later shows that the consolidation has increased throughout the right lung with the development of multiple cyst-like cavities (pneumatoceles).

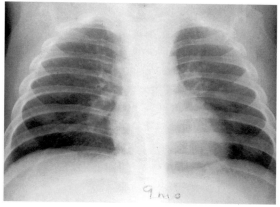

Fig. 2.65 Six months later there has been almost complete clearing of the pneumatoceles. There are a few linear densities at the hilum and the right lower lobe remains hyperlucent.

Viral pneumonias Clinically obvious viral pneumonias are less common than bacterial infections. There are three general patterns to consider.

Congenital infections – TORCH Congenital viral infection may be part of the spectrum of diseases known as TORCH (Toxoplasma, Rubella, Cytomegalovirus and Herpes). Head ultrasonography may show calcifications (see Figs 7.29, 7.30 and 7.31). 'Celery stalk' bones may be seen (see Fig. 7.32). Figure 2.66 shows generalized cardiomegaly and consolidation with air bronchograms in the left lower lung zone in a neonate with cytomegalovirus (CMV) pneumonitis.

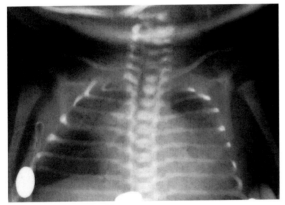

Fig. 2.66 Generalized cardiomegaly and consolidation with air bronchograms in the left lower lung zone.

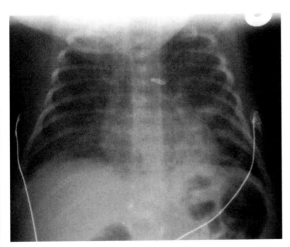

Fig. 2.67 This film of an infant with BPD was taken when the neonate was discharged from neonatal intensive care after treatment for PDA and who on discharge still had mild BPD.

Primarily respiratory illnesses Primarily respiratory illnesses, e.g. respiratory syncitial virus pneumonitis, tend to be especially seen in infants with an underlying predisposition, such as congenital heart disease or BPD, (Figs 2.67–2.69). The vector is usually the caregiver or parent, and the mode of transmission is by

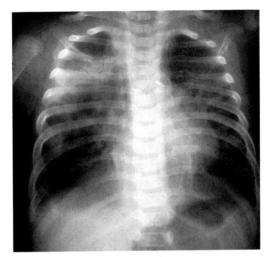

Fig. 2.68 The same infant at 6 months of age is in the acute stage of active RSV pneumonia. The changes of hyperinflation with areas of atelectasis are marked.

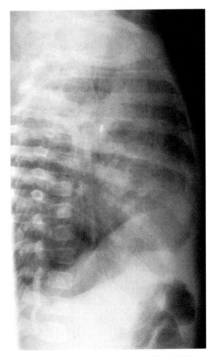

Fig. 2.69 A lateral at the same time as Fig. 2.68.

droplet spread. The differential diagnosis includes infections with other viruses, for example influenza or very rarely CMV.

Generalized enteroviral infections with cardiac failure These usually present as a form of cardiovascular collapse, often associated with acidosis. The CXR appearance is similar to cardiac failure in coarctation (Fig. 3.11). The clinical presentation is the same with profound shock. The key to differentiation is the pulses, which in myocarditis are uniformly poor, but in coarctation syndromes are discrepant between the upper and lower limbs.

PERSISTENT PULMONARY HYPERTENSION OF THE NEWBORN

Persistent pulmonary hypertension of the newborn (PPHN) results in severe hypoxaemia, and follows a poor transition to the extrauterine environment. Normally, with the first breath and the cord clamping there is a significant drop in pulmonary arterial pressure. This allows the circulation that in utero normally bypasses the lungs, to perfuse the lungs (see Fig. 8.10). In near-term infants, conditions such as cold, stress, asphyxia, aspiration syndromes, airleaks, infective conditions (especially GBS infection) and pulmonary hypoplasia do not allow this adaption to occur, and blood continues to bypass the alveoli. A further idiopathic cause is known as persistent fetal circulation; in this case the CXR shows marked oligaemia, similar to the CXR of severe pulmonary atresia. Cardiac ultrasound scans are needed to rule out congenital heart disease. The diagnosis of PPHN, however, is a clinical one, where the CXR shows the features of the primary disorder – sepsis, asphyxia, etc.

MECONIUM ASPIRATION SYNDROME

As the name implies, meconium aspiration syndrome is the result of meconium being passed in utero and then inhaled. It is caused by asphyxia, which triggers a gasping reflex and bowel motility.

Clinical features

The syndrome usually occurs in term infants, with evidence of a severe right to left shunt and severe hypoxia. The infant often has PPHN. Compounding the disease may be related features of the side-effects of therapy, i.e. severe baro-volu-trauma inflicted by hyperventilation.

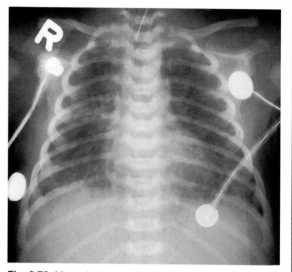

Fig. 2.70 Meconium aspiration syndrome, showing coarse, inhomogeneous deposits, particularly in the bases and perihilar areas.

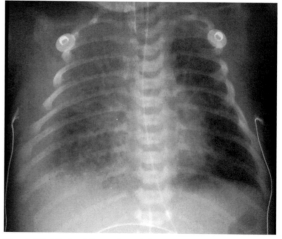

Fig. 2.71 Marked flattening of the diaphragm and overinflation, with marked bilateral infiltrates especially in the right lung. There is an associated right pleural effusion, which is not common.

Radiological appearance

Overexpanded lungs, coarse air space consolidation, and pneumothorax or pneumomediastinum are typical findings in meconium aspiration syndrome (Figs 2.70–2.72).

AMNIOTIC FLUID ASPIRATION

Amniotic fluid aspiration is usually less severe than meconium aspiration syndrome. It characteristically results from inhalation of 'squames' and leads to a horrific CXR appearance which may be far worse than the picture of the infant clinically.

Radiological appearance

Overexpanded lungs with poorly defined, hazy density, which usually improve rapidly, are typical findings (Figs 2.73, 2.74).

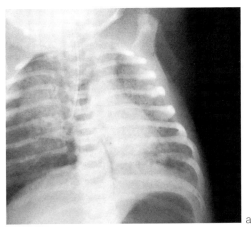

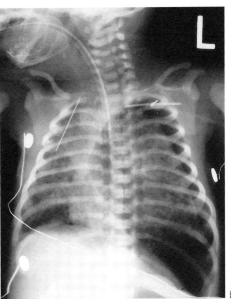

Fig. 2.72 Two films taken 8 days apart in the same patient. The first film (a) shows coarse, inhomogeneous deposits. Film (b) taken 8 days later shows marked hyperinflation due to air trapping with flattening of the diaphragms. A tension pneumothorax has developed on the left with shifting of the mediastinum to the right.

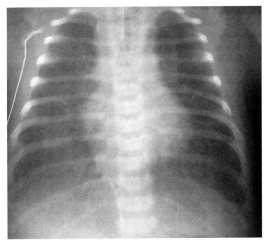

Fig. 2.73 Amniotic fluid aspiration. This film shows bilateral diffuse fine to coarse interstitial markings. The differential diagnosis includes pneumonia and TTN; the latter is less likely as no fluid-filled fissure is apparent.

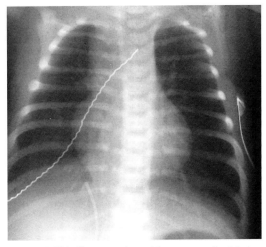

Fig. 2.74 This film was taken of the same patient 1 day after Fig. 2.73 and shows clearing of the lungs. There is still mild overexpansion as seen by the interstitial bulging between the ribs.

PULMONARY HYPOPLASIA

Underdeveloped lungs can result from many underlying causes. Two of these causes are detailed below and three others are contained in the section Surgical problems in the chest (p. 42 and Figs 2.85–2.87).

- Presentation: depending on its severity, pulmonary hypoplasia may be obvious in the delivery room, with hypoxia and hypercapnia. The difficulty in resuscitation may mimic birth asphyxia, and high ventilatory pressures may be needed. Later presentations include persistent pulmonary hypertension and airleak syndromes. Sometimes a malformed chest may be present. Specific antenatal features may include prolonged rupture of membranes or other causes of oligaemia.
- General CXR features: there is a wide spectrum of radiographic appearances on CXR depending on the aetiology, with a common feature of small lungs.

Oligohydramnios sequence

Clinical features The combination of skeletal contractures, oligohydramnios, anuria or oliguria, severe perinatal asphyxia is known as Potter's sequence or syndrome. This syndrome results in pulmonary hypoplasia as a result of decreased amniotic fluid and the consequent increased pressure on the fetal chest in utero.

Radiological appearance An ultrasound scan is helpful to distinguish complete renal agenesis (where the prognosis is hopeless) from pseudo-Potter's syndrome (oligohydramnios with some degree of renal function) where the prognosis is less certain (Fig. 2.75).

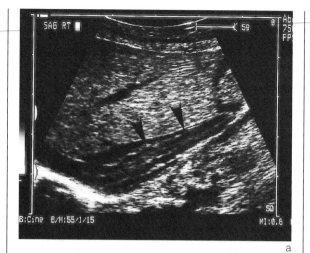

a

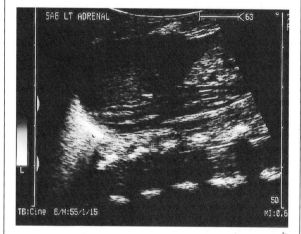

b

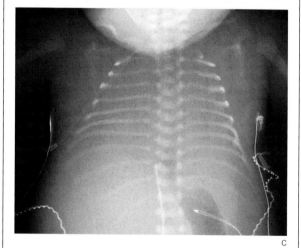

c

Fig. 2.75 Ultrasound images of a neonate showing a bilateral renal agenesis in a patient with Potter's syndrome; arrows show renal bed with only adrenals present (a, b). A chest film from another neonate (c) with pulmonary hypoplasia shows the typically small thorax.

Neuromuscular disorders

Clinical features Apnoea with neuromuscular fatigue and floppiness is typical, with ventilator dependency. The history may include maternal drug ingestion (phenytoin), polyhydramnios, decreased fetal movements, and maternal myotonic dystrophy, myasthenia gravis, etc.

Radiological appearance Figure 2.76 shows a neonate whose mother had previously unsuspected myotonic dystrophy. Note the small lung volumes (in spite of the patient being intubated) and the high diaphragms. Also note the thin ribs typical of myotonic dystrophy. Ribs vary in thickness and density: there are poorly mineralized and thin ribs, and some extremely thin ones which are widely separated, as a result of poorly developed intercostal muscles. Diaphragms are high especially on the right. The heart is large and globular.

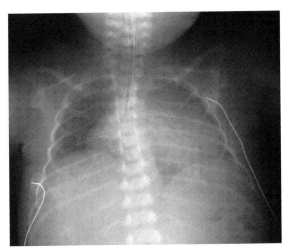

Fig. 2.76 Neonate with maternal myotonic dystrophy (see text).

PLEURAL EFFUSIONS

Clinical features

The clinical features depend upon the time of presentation, i.e. whether the condition is congenital or acquired. Many congenital cases present in the delivery room or in the hours following birth; these present with respiratory failure and have associated features of polyhydramnios or hydrops fetalis syndromes. Emergency drainage of the pleural effusion and possibly also of the ascites may be required.

A later presentation may follow feeding, resulting in chylothorax. These cases may also present in the delivery room with respiratory distress and pleural fluid. The pleural effusion contains chylomicrons on examination if feeds have been given. In some, a history may be obtained of a rupture of the thoracic chyle ducts – that is to say a traumatic delivery with a history of rotational injury. Some chylothoraces follow thoracic surgery, most commonly for patent ductus arteriosus, where ligation may traumatize the ducts. Also following any thoracic surgery, fluid accumulation is frequent (see for example cystic adenomatoid malformation, Fig. 2.83).

Management is to delay surgical treatment, in the hope that new channels of lymph absorption will spontaneously develop. Some cases will not resolve, and in these difficult and often protracted scenarios pleural stripping may be undertaken. Total parenteral nutrition (TPN) is required since enteral feeding exacerbates the problem. However, feeds with medium chain triglycerides (Portagen) formula may allow enteral feeding without reaccumulation of the chylothorax. For persistent chylothorax, mass ligation of the thoracic duct can be performed at the level of the diaphragm via a right or left thoracotomy.

Pleural effusions secondary to infections are usually small and resolve with the treatment of the underlying infection.

Radiological appearance

Fluid is most apparent at the costophrenic angles. However, since most neonatal films are taken with the infant lying supine, small amounts of fluid are often missed. Moreover, fluid may appear at the apex.

Figure 2.77 shows a pleural effusion complicating a case of group B streptococcal pneumonia. There is a small to moderate pleural effusion on the right. The lungs are well expanded but show some consolidation at the bases. The left lung shows some compensatory hyperexpansion. Hypoxia has necessitated IPPV and oxygen. For other examples of pleural effusions from GBS infection, see section on pneumonia.

Figure 2.78 is a film of a 3-day-old neonate showing a massive right-sided pleural effusion with shift of the mediastinum to the left, due to chylothorax. The infant had undergone a difficult birth with a double footling breech presentation and forceps delivery. The infant at the time the film was taken was pale but without apparent respiratory distress. After placement of a chest tube and feeding with infant formula it was noted that the originally clear pleural fluid turned milky, confirming a chylothorax. The

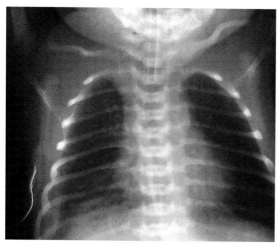

Fig. 2.77 Pleural effusion in group B streptococcal pneumonia.

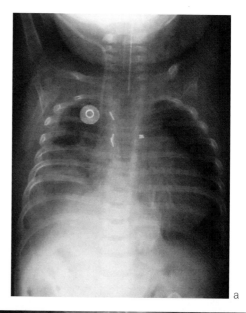

a

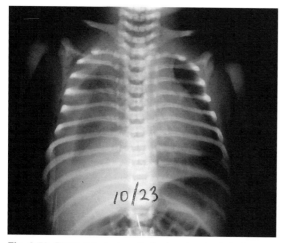

Fig. 2.78 Right-sided pleural effusion due to chylothorax in a 3-day-old neonate.

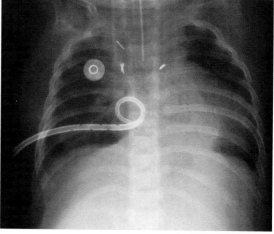

b

Fig. 2.79 Primary chylothorax: (a) presentation; (b) post-thoracotomy drainage, with a pigtail catheter.

child did well after chest tube drainage and was sent home. Follow-up examinations showed complete resolution.

Figure 2.79 illustrates a primary chylothorax not heralded by any birth abnormality. The infant was treated with long-term TPN and then with medium-chain triglycerides. Note also the abdominal distension with evidence of fluid.

Figure 2.80 is a series of films demonstrating the development of a postoperative chylothorax after surgical

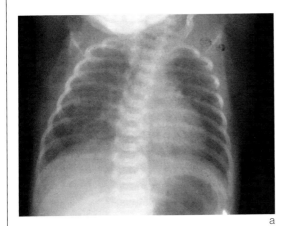

a

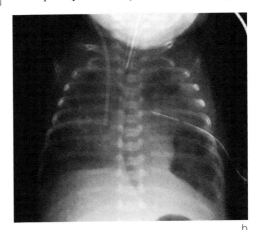

b

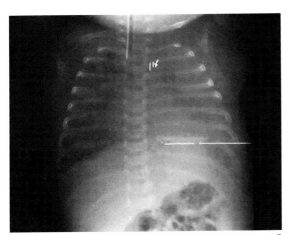

c

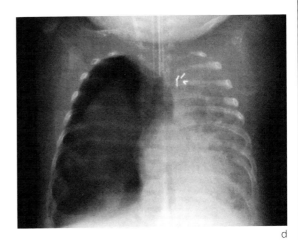

d

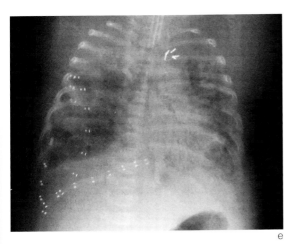

e

Fig. 2.80 Development of postoperative chylothorax. On day 1 of life (a), the film was normal. On day 27 of life, a few days after surgical ligation of the PDA, the film shows diffuse severe lung disease (b) with a large left pleural effusion which proved to be a chylothorax. On day 62, again a large left pleural effusion is seen (c). New surgical clips are seen from an unsuccessful attempt to clip oozing mediastinal lymphatic vessels. Diffuse lung disease is also visible. On day 73(d) a tension pneumothorax is seen on the right. The chylous pleural effusion is again noted on the left. On day 78(e) there is diffuse bilateral extensive lung disease with bilateral pleural effusions. Note the pleuroperitoneal shunt that has been placed in an attempt to drain the recurrent pleural effusions.

ligation of PDA. A pleuroperitoneal shunt was eventually placed in an attempt to drain the recurrent pleural effusions, but this extreme measure was unsuccessful and the patient died that day from respiratory deterioration.

Fig. 2.81 is another example of a patient with a massive right chylous pleural effusion secondary to birth trauma. The first film shows almost complete opacification of the right hemithorax. A second film taken 2 weeks later after drainage of the effusion still shows a significant amount of pleural fluid remaining. However, in this case spontaneous full resolution occurred allowing drain removal and feeding by the normal route to be established.

PULMONARY HAEMORRHAGE

In pulmonary haemorrhage there is bleeding from the airway, usually accompanied by respiratory insufficiency. It can be a dramatic event; the spectrum may range from a small amount of blood in the trachea, to increased respiratory distress and a moderate amount of fresh blood, to complete cardiovascular collapse with massive bleeding. There are three main causes:

1. Sudden and major opening of a PDA may result in dramatically increased left to right shunt with massive pulmonary haemorrhage. Indomethacin is contraindicated and emergency duct ligation may be needed.
2. With a history of asphyxia, myocardial failure may be present. An electrocardiogram may document ischaemia.
3. Sometimes following surfactant treatment the pulmonary vascular resistance may rapidly drop, leading to vascular engorgement with haemorrhage. Paradoxically, surfactant can treat the resultant respiratory failure because the haemorrhage reduces the surface-active properties of the surfactant, and this may need further boosting.

The differential diagnosis includes trauma, disseminated intravascular coagulation and congenital malformations. All are unusual causes of this type of problem.

Figure 2.82 shows the radiographic features of pulmonary haemorrhage over the course of a week in a preterm infant.

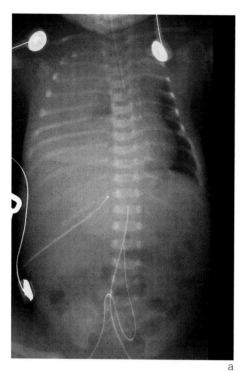

a

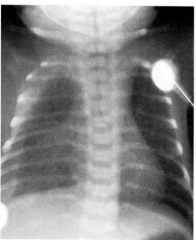

b

Fig. 2.81 Massive chylous pleural effusion secondary to birth trauma. (a) There is almost complete opacification of the right hemithorax. (b) Two weeks later after drainage of the effusion a significant amount of pleural fluid remains.

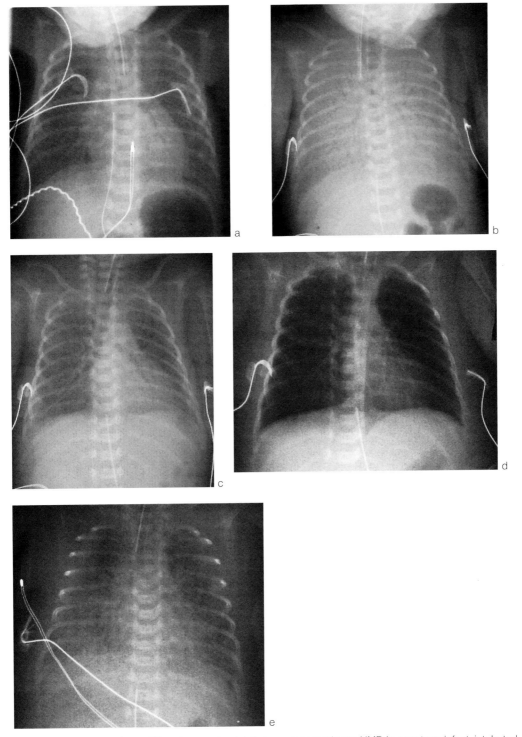

Fig. 2.82 Pulmonary haemorrhage. Film taken on day 1 (a) shows only moderate HMD in a preterm infant, intubated during the first day of life. This was treated successfully with surfactant. On day 2, a marked deterioration associated with a pulmonary haemorrhage was found (b). The CXR shows a 'white-out' pattern of bilateral increased densities. Increased positive end-expiratory pressure (PEEP) therapy led to an improvement, as shown by films taken on day 3 (c) and day 4 (d). On day 7 of life, an attempted extubation was followed by a massive haemorrhage, and the CXR (e) showed a return of the previous appearance of bilateral pulmonary densities. This infant did not survive.

SURGICAL PROBLEMS IN THE CHEST

Compression syndrome: space-occupying lesion in the thorax

Clinical features The diagnosis includes space-occupying lesions in the lung itself: congenital cystic adenomatoid malformation (CCAM), cystic hygroma and tumour.

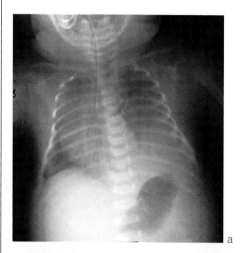

a

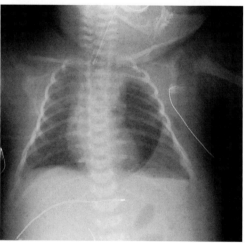

b

Fig. 2.83 Two films taken before (a) and after (b) surgery for congenital cystic adenomatoid malformation. Note the ill-defined density in the left lower hemithorax causing a mass effect with shift of the mediastinum and heart to the right (a). The postoperative film shows a more normal position of the heart (b). A residual postoperative pleural effusion remains. The differential diagnosis for the original findings in (a) would include pulmonary sequestration and diaphragmatic hernia. Sequestrations present with masses, only rarely in the newborn, and then are usually extra-lobar. Intra-lobar sequestrations present later in life, unless associated with cardiac malformations.

Radiological appearance Figure 2.83 shows the appearance of CCAM before and after surgery. Figure 2.84 illustrates a chest teratoma.

Congenital chest deformities

There are several congenital skeletal abnormalities that lead to a very small thorax and associated *pulmonary hypoplasia*. Perhaps the most severe are the skeletal anomalies of Jeune's syndrome (asphyxiating thoracic dystrophy) and osteogenesis imperfecta, (Figs 2.85, 2.86). Some of these lead to very early death, but this is not invariable (see Chapter 7).

Diaphragmatic hernia

Congenital diaphragmatic hernia is caused by failure of closure of the pleuroperitoneal fold by the 9th week of gestational age. Associated anomalies in 20% effect the central nervous system (neural tube defects), gastrointestinal tract (malrotation, oral cleft, omphalocele), and cardiovascular and genitourinary systems. Herniated organs include the small bowel, stomach, large bowel, spleen, pancreas, kidney and liver.

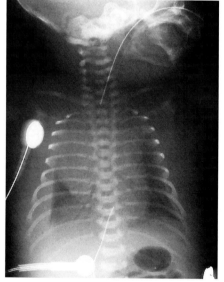

Fig. 2.84 Teratoma in chest with hydrops. This AP view shows an ill-defined density in the upper thorax. Note the significantly thickened soft tissues over the chest (hydrops).

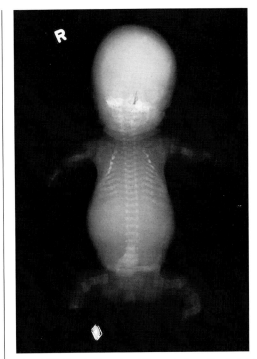

Fig. 2.85 Single film of a stillborn baby with skeletal findings of osteogenesis imperfecta. These findings include thick, malformed long bones resulting from multiple fractures in utero and poor ossification of the cranium. Note the small, bell-shaped thorax resulting from pulmonary hypoplasia, another finding in osteogenesis imperfecta.

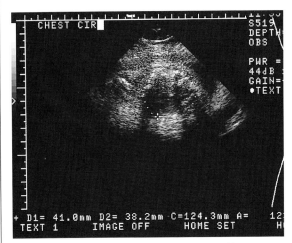

Fig. 2.86 Osteogenesis imperfecta diagnosed in utero with a very small thorax on US. The prognosis was given as hopeless. The single US image of the fetal chest shows a chest circumference corresponding to an estimated gestational age of 19 weeks. The chronological age was 26 weeks.

Clinical features Clinical presentation is respiratory distress which may occur in the delivery room, with failure to respond to resuscitation. Both survival and age of presentation depend upon the degree of *pulmonary hypoplasia*, which in turn depends upon the gestational age at which the hernia occurred. Clinically PPHN is often marked, and may prompt treatment with high frequency oscillation, extracorporeal membrane oxygenation or nitric oxide.

Radiological appearance The CXR is a poor guide to the degree of hypoplasia. Figure 2.87 shows two films of a baby who presented with late respiratory distress at 4 days old. In the

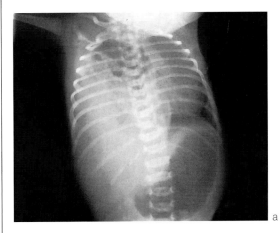

a

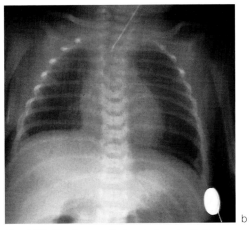

b

Fig. 2.87 Diaphragmatic hernia (see text). On presentation at 4 days of age (a) the lung appears severely compromised; however, 4 days postoperatively (b) the lung shows only mild hypoplasia, if any.

first film the right hemidiaphragm is not visible and there is a density in the right lower chest area with cystic areas in the lung apex. The stomach is below the diaphragm but the atrium is shifted to the right and is distended. The mediastinum is to the left with corresponding expansion only of the left lung base. There is probably bowel and liver in the right chest. From this film the lung appears severely compromised, but the degree of hypoplasia is uncertain. However, in the film taken 4 days after surgery, the lung shows only mild hypoplasia, if any.

Figures 2.88–2.90 show a series of films from a second infant with a later presentation. This late form of presentation may be truly congenital, or may be acquired following a group B streptococcal disease. Presumably the latter induces some myopathic change in the hemidiaphragm. Both causes are usually evident on the right side rather than the left. Ultrasonography may be helpful when this is suspected.

An even further delayed presentation is shown in a 6-week-old infant who presented in extremis (Fig. 2.91). The differential diagnosis includes cystic malformation of the lung, lobar emphysema and staphylococcal pneumatocele, and if one notices the absence

of the stomach below the diaphragm one thinks of congenital diaphragmatic hernia, which is what this is.

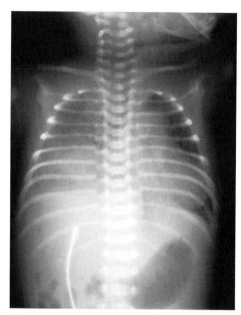

Fig. 2.89 In the same patient as in Fig. 2.88, film taken 1 day later shows a mass in the right lower hemithorax.

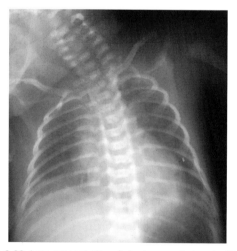

Fig. 2.88 Late presentation of diaphragmatic hernia. This film taken a few days after birth shows indistinctness of the right hemidiaphragm only.

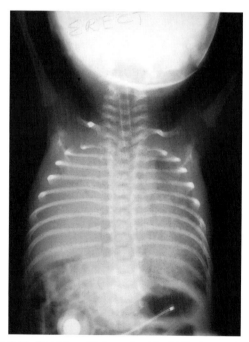

Fig. 2.90 Film taken 10 days after Fig. 2.89, shows a large mass from a right diaphragmatic hernia occupying the whole right hemithorax and causing a mass effect with deviation of the mediastinum to the left.

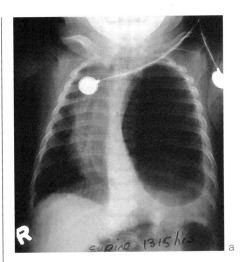

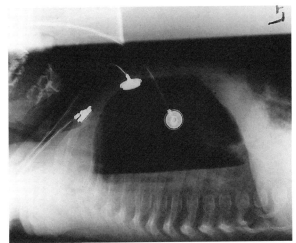

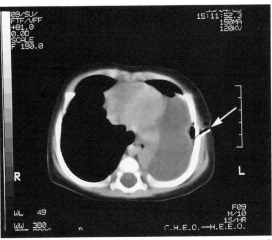

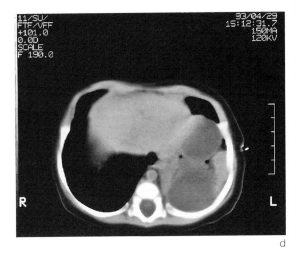

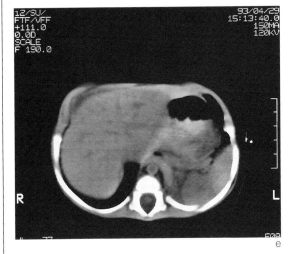

Fig. 2.91 Diaphragmatic hernia presenting at 6 weeks of age. A huge cystic mass (a) can be seen entirely filling the left hemithorax and shifting the mediastinum to the right. Because of fulminant respiratory distress, the left chest was aspirated under the impression that it was a pneumothorax. A chest tube was placed which did not drain much (see arrow in CT image (c)). The stomach in the chest shows up in the CT images as fluid filled. The lateral view (b) shows it is partially filled with fluid. Films (c) to (e) show a sequence of CT images which still demonstrates a loop of dilated stomach within the left hemithorax in the high cuts (c to d) and then liver in the low cut (e) on the right.

Double aortic arch

Anomalies of the great vessels usually present with stridor, sometimes with repeated vomiting and cyanosis. The infant in Figure 2.92 had stridor, prompting suspicion of a vascular ring which was first diagnosed at bronchoscopy. This was followed by a barium swallow which showed the characteristic appearance of a posterior indentation of the oesophagus indicating a vascular ring. This infant had a double aortic arch.

Bronchogenic cyst

The neonate in Figure 2.93 presented with respiratory distress and expiratory stridor. The AP film is unremarkable but the lateral CXR clearly shows the separation of the trachea and the oesophagus. A CT scan of the chest demonstrated the cystic nature of this mediastinal lesion.

Lobar emphysema

The CXR in a 1-day-old infant with respiratory distress clearly shows a hyperlucent left upper lobe seen in lobar emphysema (Fig. 2.94). This was treated with lobectomy with complete resolution of symptoms.

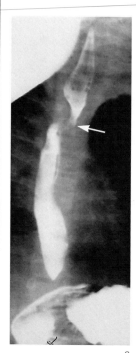 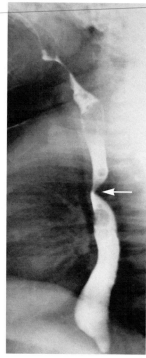

a   b

Fig. 2.92 Double aortic arch. Bronchoscopy suggested the presence of a vascular ring. (a) AP view of the oesophagus during upper gastrointestinal swallow study, with displacement of contrast column in the upper thorax from the vascular ring (arrow). (b) Appearance of a posterior indentation of the oesophagus (arrow).

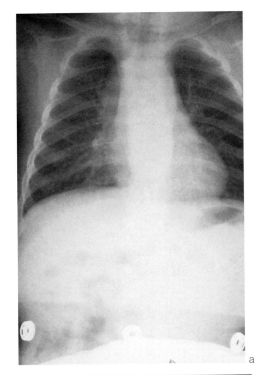

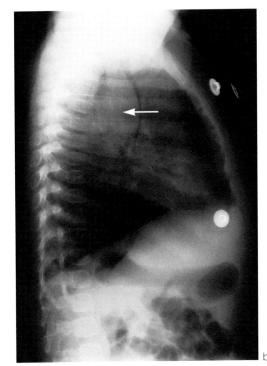

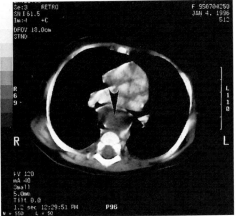

Fig. 2.93 Bronchogenic cyst. The AP film (a) appears normal but the lateral view (b) shows the separation of the trachea and the oesophagus (arrow). The cystic nature of the lesion is demonstrated by CT (c). This should measure 0–5 Hounsfield units.

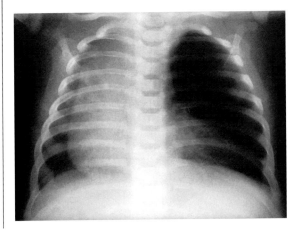

Fig. 2.94 Lobar emphysema (see text).

Bronchial stenosis

The neonate in Figure 2.95 had multiple anomalies including oesophageal atresia, congenital heart disease and bronchial stenosis.

Congenital cystic adenomatoid malformation

An example of congenital cystic adenomatoid malformation (CCAM) is shown in Figure 2.96.

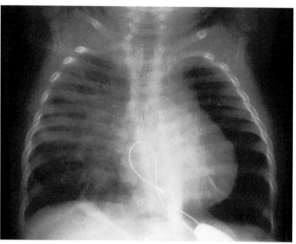
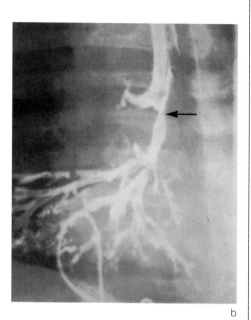

a b

Fig. 2.95 Bronchial stenosis in a neonate with multiple anomalies. (a) Chronic changes in the right lung field, especially in the lower lung field. Cardiac pacing wires are seen. (b) Bronchogram with water-soluble contrast demonstrating a stricture (arrow) in the bronchus intermedius just below the take-off of the right upper lobe bronchus.

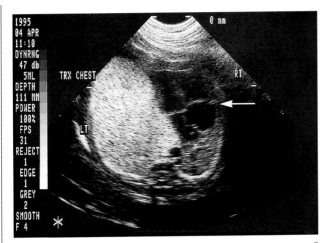

a

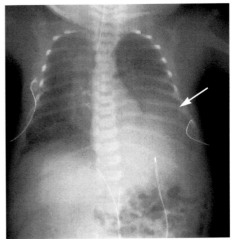

b

c

Fig. 2.96 Antenatal ultrasound scan (a) defines an echogenic right chest mass at the level of the heart and stomach (transverse image – heart arrow) and located posteriorly. The CXR findings (b) were subtle with only a 'soft tissue' effect (arrow) which obscures the leaf of the diaphragm on the left, but the CT scan (c) of the neonate's chest helped define the cystic mass and its location.

References

Bancalari E, Abdenour G E, Feller R, Gannon J 1979 Bronchopulmonary dysplasia: clinical presentation. Journal of Pediatrics 95: 819–823

Kirpalani H, Coblentz C, Monkman S et al 1977. Computer aided measurement of lung volume from chest X-ray. Paediatric Research 41(4): 257A

Krauss A V, Klain D B, Auld P A 1975 Chronic pulmonary insufficiency of prematurity (CPIP). Pediatrics 55: 55–58

Northway W H, Rosan R C, Porter D Y 1974 Pulmonary disease following respirator therapy of hyaline membrane disease. New England Journal of Medicine 276: 357–368

Shennan A T, Dunn M S, Ohlsson A, Lennox K, Hoskins E M, 1988 Abnormal pulmonary outcomes in premature infants: prediction from oxygen requirement in the neonatal period. Pediatrics 82: 527–532

Stringel G, Mercer S, Bass J 1984 Surgical management of persistent postoperative chylothorax in children. Canadian Journal of Surgery, vol 27, 6: 543–546

Tudor J, Young L, Wigglesworth J S, Steiner R E 1976 The value of radiology in the idiopathic respiratory distress syndrome: a radiological and pathological correlation study. Clinical Radiology 27: 65–75

Weinstein M R, Peters M E, Sadek M, Palta M 1995 A new radiographic scoring system for BPD. Pediatric Pulmonology 18: 284–289

Wilson M E, Mikity V E 1960 A new form of respiratory disease in premature infants. American Journal of Diseases of Children 99: 489–499

CHAPTER 3

Congenital heart lesions

Haresh Kirpalani
John Mernagh
Gerald Gill

CLASSIFICATION

Congenital heart lesions should be classified clinically into cyanotic or acyanotic lesions, which forms the starting point for interpreting the radiological findings.

- Cyanotic lesions are usually subdivided into those with decreased pulmonary vascularity (oligaemia) and those with increased pulmonary vascularity (plethora). Disorders with plethora include transposition of the great arteries, truncus arteriosus, severe ventricular defects with oedema, total anomalous pulmonary venous return, and single ventricle. Disorders with oligaemia include tetralogy of Fallot, simple pulmonary stenosis or atresia (or complex lesions with stenosis, e.g. transposition with pulmonary stenosis and ventricular septal defect (VSD), or double outlet ventricle with pulmonary stenosis and VSD), tricuspid atresia, and Ebstein's anomaly.
- Acyanotic lesions are generally the left to right shunts that produce pulmonary plethora or increased flow (such as atrial septal defect, VSD and patent ductus arteriosus), or cardiac failure from lesions such as coarctation of the aorta.

PRESENTATION OF CONGENITAL HEART DISEASE

Clinical presentation

The clinical situation faced is usually one of a baby who is hypoxaemic; a baby in heart failure; or a baby who is ventilator-dependent.

The general approach is to distinguish between respiratory disease and cardiac disease. Since the infant is often suspected of having respiratory distress syndrome (RDS), the infant may be treated with surfactant. If the hypoxaemia resolves, this will require no further investigation. However, if the infant is still hypoxaemic or ventilator-dependent or has heart failure, it is essential that a full clinical examination including synchrony of pulses and blood pressure and a hyperoxic test are performed. Also, consider whether the chest X-ray (CXR) is unduly 'plethoric' or unduly 'oligaemic'. A cardiac ultrasound scan may be needed urgently.

Radiological features

1. *Oligaemia.* Decreased pulmonary vascularity in 'lucent' lungs – i.e. 'black' lungs with few vascular markings – can be confused with either hyperinflation or pneumothorax. Look for small, tapered vessels. In pneumothorax there is usually a margin which can be seen representing the edge of collapsed lung. In oligaemia, although the tapered vessels cannot be traced to the lung margin, this occupies the whole thorax.
2. *Plethora.* There is an increase in the size and number of visible pulmonary vessels, extending more to the periphery of the lungs and evenly distributed throughout the lungs. A redistribution between the upper and lower lung zones as seen in adults in cardiac failure does not apply.

Some classic radiological presentations are considered below. We emphasize that these 'rules' are often broken, especially in complex lesions.

Cyanosis with oligaemia Figures 3.1–3.5 show five examples of cyanotic neonates with oligaemic lungs.

Figure 3.1 shows the characteristic signs of the tetralogy of Fallot. Note the rounded, upturned apex of the heart indicative of right ventricular (RV) hypertrophy. Note also the

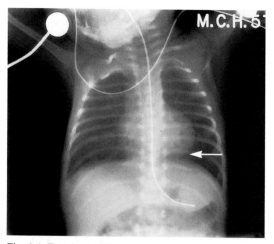

Fig. 3.1 Tetralogy of Fallot, showing the typical upturned cardiac apex lifted off the diaphragm (arrow) and oligaemic lungs.

decreased lung vascularity due to the pulmonary stenosis. It should be noted that the RV hypertrophy is progressive and thus newborns may not have an upturned apex. Figure 3.2 shows an example of tetralogy of Fallot before and after a Blalock procedure (a surgical shunt between the pulmonary artery and the subclavian artery). The first film shows a typical picture of tetralogy of Fallot with an upturned cardiac apex and oligaemic lungs. This patient also had a right-sided aortic arch (arrow). The same patient is shown after the Blalock procedure showing the significantly improved pulmonary vascularity. Associated with this is an increased cardiac size. Ebstein's anomaly is associated with a huge heart and decreased pulmonary vascularity (Fig. 3.3). The cardiomegaly is often extreme, and one differential diagnosis includes myocarditis. The electrocardiograph in Ebstein's anomaly should show left axis deviation (LAD) and in myocarditis there are inverted T waves. Myocarditis also has pulmonary plethora on CXR.

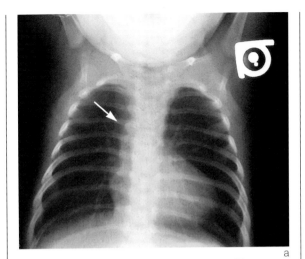

a

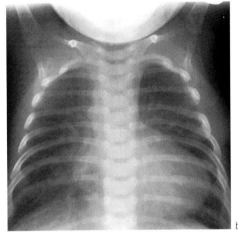

b

Fig. 3.2 Tetralogy of Fallot (a) before and (b) after Blalock's procedure. There is also a right-sided aortic arch (arrowed).

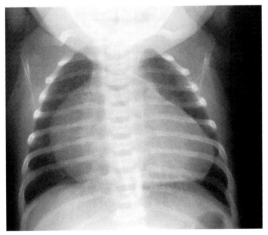

Fig. 3.3 Ebstein's anomaly showing cardiomegaly and decreased pulmonary vascularity.

Other cyanotic conditions with oligaemia are lesions with a predominant impediment to pulmonary flow as in more complex lesions such as transposition of the great arteries with pulmonary atresia (Fig. 3.4) and asplenia complex with pulmonary atresia (Fig. 3.5).

Cyanosis with plethora Figures 3.6 and 3.7 show two examples of cyanotic neonates with increased pulmonary vascularity.

Acyanosis with heart failure Figures 3.8 and 3.9 show two examples of acyanotic neonates with increased pulmonary vascularity. Figure 3.8 shows a VSD and Figure 3.9 shows a late presentation of a patent ductus arteriosus (PDA).

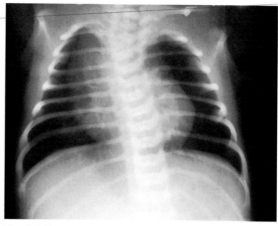

Fig. 3.4 Transposition of the great arteries with pulmonary atresia. Note the oligaemic lungs. There are also vertebral anomalies in the upper thoracic spine.

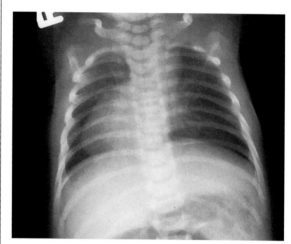

Fig. 3.5 Asplenia complex. This patient showed dextrocardia, oligaemic lungs and a midline liver. At autopsy a single atrium, a single ventricle of left ventricular morphology with a single atrioventricular valve of mitral morphology, and pulmonary atresia were found.

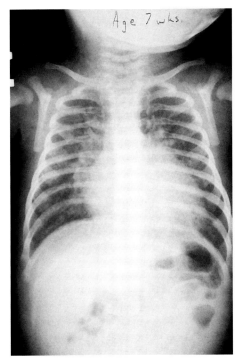

Fig. 3.6 Transposition of the great arteries with VSD. Note the increased pulmonary vascularity, especially in comparison with Fig. 3.4.

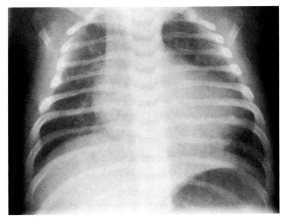

Fig. 3.7 Truncus arteriosus. Again note the increased pulmonary vascularity.

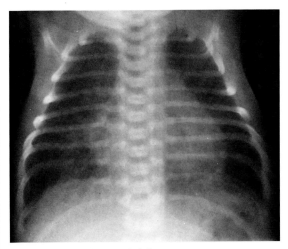

Fig. 3.8 Ventricular septal defect.

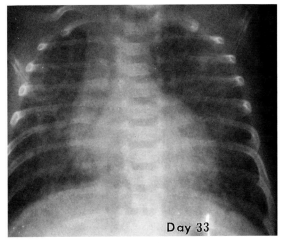

Fig. 3.9 Patent ductus arteriosus.

Figures 3.10 and 3.11 show two examples of neonates in congestive failure. The degree of congestive failure may confer significant cyanosis to the presentation. Distinguishing failure from plethora is a clinical not radiological task. The indistinctness of the heart and pulmonary vessels as seen in these images is indicative of failure. Figure 3.11 consists of two images from before and after surgery of an acyanotic neonate who was admitted to hospital 10 days after birth. The child had had an uneventful delivery and was discharged home, but returned in failure. This type of dramatic presentation of shock in an infant may be due to myocarditis, severe sepsis or inborn error of metabolism. This patient, however, had preductal coarctation of the aorta. This is typically diagnosed by absent pulses and cardiac failure. The postoperative film is essentially normal.

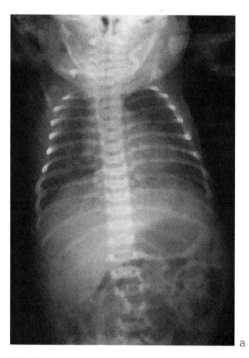

a

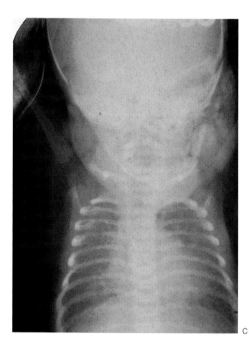

c

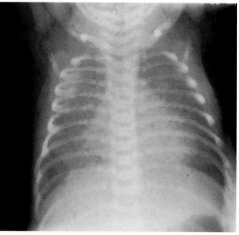

b

Fig. 3.10 Three images taken at days 3, 6, 9 days of life respectively in a moderately cyanotic neonate. Note the progressive worsening of the failure with no progressive increase in heart size. This is indicative of total anomalous pulmonary venous return below the diaphragm (causing obstruction), the diagnosis in this case.

More bizarre forms of cardiac failure may involve high-output failure not of primarily cardiac origin. The 36-week-old infant in Figure 3.12 presented at birth with respiratory distress, tachycardia, hepatomegaly and ascites. Diagnosis was high-output cardiac failure secondary to hepatic haemangioma. The infant was ventilated and treated with digoxin, a diuretic and steroids, but died at 72 hours of age. The film shows generalized cardiomegaly and gross hepatomegaly, with a distended abdomen and displacement of the stomach and upper small bowel gas to the left side. (See also Figure 5.23)

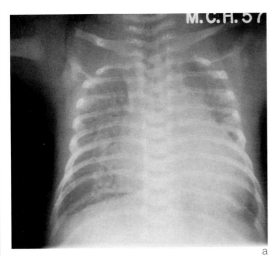

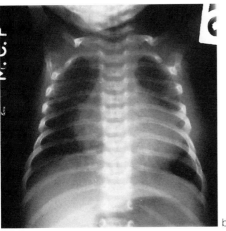

Fig. 3.11 Neonatal congestive heart failure, due to preductal coarctation of the aorta (see text). (a) Before surgery; (b) after surgery.

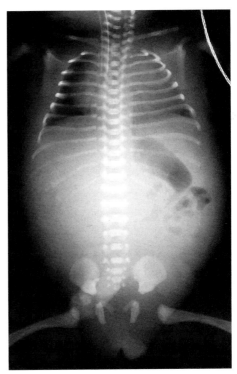

Fig. 3.12 Generalized cardiomegaly and gross hepatomegaly in an infant with high-output cardiac failure secondary to hepatic haemangioma; note the intraabdominal gas all pushed laterally. (N.B. The ETT is too low.)

METABOLIC HEART DISEASE WITH FAILURE

Hypothyroidism and hyperthyroidism

Hypothyroidism and hyperthyroidism both can present in the newborn with heart failure. The clinical features that distinguish the two entities revolve around the ancillary features of tremors, staring gaze, hyperreflexia and wasting in the thyrotoxic infant; and hypotonia, hypoglycaemia and hypothermia in the hypothyroid infant.

On X-ray examination cardiomegaly is seen in both hypothyroidism (Fig. 3.13) and hyperthyroidism (Fig. 3.14).

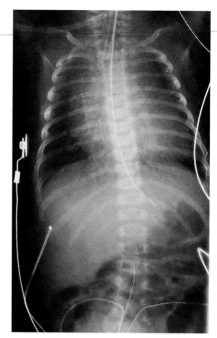

Fig. 3.13 Generalized cardiomegaly of hypothyroidism.

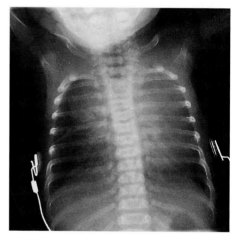

Fig. 3.14 An AP film of a neonate with hyperthyroidism. There is cardiomegaly with signs of failure (i.e. interstitial and pleural fluid).

Hypoglycaemia and infants of diabetic mothers

Infants of diabetic mothers can have cardiomegaly. In these infants hypertrophic obstructive cardiomyopathy may be seen. An example is shown in Chapter 2 (see Fig. 2.15).

Even without a history of maternal diabetes, hypoglycaemia can cause cardiac dilatation, but usually resolves as hypoglycaemia is controlled. Figure 3.15 shows a more intractable form of hypoglycaemia associated with nesidioblastosis, a tumour-like condition of type II islet cells, which may result in mental retardation unless adequately treated. This mandates early surgical placement of long intravenous lines to allow access for glucose replacement. This infant illustrates the severe associated cardiac dilatation. Figure 3.15 shows films taken on presentation and 1 month later, showing deterioration despite the administration of steroids and diazoxide therapy. It is important to exclude type II glycogen storage disorders (Pompe's disease) which may mandate biopsy of the liver or heart. If nesidioblastosis is confirmed a subtotal pancreatectomy may be required.

References

Freedom R M, Benson L N, Smallhorn J F (eds) 1992 Neonatal heart disease. Springer-Verlag, Berlin

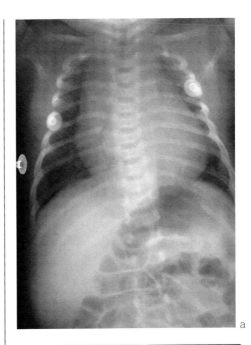

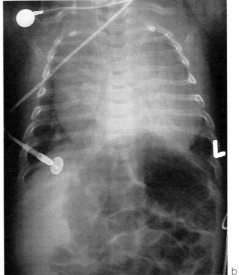

Fig. 3.15 Two films from a subject with nesidioblastosis. Initially there is only mild generalized cardiomegaly without hepatomegaly (a). One month later (b) there is gross cardiomegaly with signs of failure. There is a central venous line into the right atrium.

CHAPTER 4

The abdomen

Mark Walton
Gerald Gill
John Mernagh
Haresh Kirpalani

INTRODUCTION

Air as a contrast agent

In evaluating the gastrointestinal (GI) tract in the neonate, the plain film of the chest and abdomen is the most useful first radiographic examination. Infants swallow air virtually with the first breath so that the GI tract, usually within the first few hours of postnatal life, contains air from the stomach to the rectum. However, the distinctive patterns allowing one to distinguish between small bowel and colon, seen in older children and adults, are not apparent in the neonate; in the normal neonatal plain abdominal film one sees gas in the stomach and in the rest of the bowel without distinguishing between small bowel and colon. Other abdominal organs such as the liver and a full bladder are seen only as they displace gas-filled loops of bowel. On plain films of the chest the oesophagus occasionally can be seen.

The normal air in the neonatal GI tract is a useful contrast medium, permitting diagnosis of many congenital anomalies without the use of barium or other contrast media given by mouth, nasogastric tube or enema. For example, in oesophageal atresia the upper pouch is often distended with air and can be seen on a plain film. The presence or absence of a fistula from the trachea to the oesophagus is determined by the presence or absence of air in the stomach and bowel.

In left-sided diaphragmatic hernia, air in bowel in the left chest may not be present in the initial film but usually is apparent in subsequent films. The absence of air in the normal locations (stomach and jejunum) on an early film with a gasless left chest are useful diagnostic signs. With right-sided diaphragmatic hernia there may be only liver in the right chest on initial films simulating hypoplasia of the right lung, atelectasis or consolidation, but the presence of gas-filled loops in the normal anatomic location of the liver can be the clue that the liver is in the chest.

The traditional signs of duodenal atresia, 'double bubble', and jejunal atresia, 'triple bubble', are reliable signs on early plain films. Obstructions and atresias further down the GI tract may not be as reliably diagnosed on early films but later, as air reaches the obstruction, the number of loops distended with air roughly corresponds to the level of atresia and estimates of upper, mid or lower small bowel obstruction may be made on the plain film.

Contrast GI examinations

Barium has been the traditional contrast agent for GI studies. It is cheap, readily available, provides good contrast and is inert, but its disadvantages in the neonate are the dangers of aspiration, and the risk that it may form solid clumps in the bowel above an obstruction or with meconium ileus. In cases of a perforation the barium remains in the peritoneal cavity, is very difficult to remove and may form granulomas until removed by a surgeon.

Non-ionic or low-osmolar water-soluble contrast is frequently used today in neonates. With this type of contrast, aspiration may still cause increased respiratory distress, but the formation of solid clumps in the bowel is not a problem and if perforations are present the contrast is absorbed by the peritoneum and excreted by the kidneys. Indeed the appearance of contrast in the urinary tract may be the initial sign confirming that a perforation has occurred.

Frequently a decision must be made in suspected intestinal obstruction as to whether an upper GI or a contrast enema is the most appropriate study. If the obstruction is thought to be high in the intestine, e.g. duodenal stenosis, annular pancreas, malrotation or jejunal atresia, then an upper GI study may be appropriate and give a timely diagnosis. Where more distal small bowel problems are suspected, an enema contrast study quickly establishes that there is a small, 'unused' colon, and contrast may reflux into the terminal ileum, also 'unused', and occasionally may reach the level of obstruction. This usually gives sufficient evidence for the surgeon. Attempting to reach a distal small bowel obstruction with contrast delivered to the stomach is often time-consuming, and contrast is diluted by fluid in the distended loops of bowel with unrewarding results.

NEONATAL GASTROINTESTINAL OBSTRUCTION

Obstruction can result at a number of anatomical sites secondary to extraluminal, intraluminal or intramural causes that occlude forward passage of enteral contents.

General appearance

Clinical features Most of the atresias are thought to result in utero from vascular accidents in the mesentery. The level of obstruction will dictate presentation.

- Oesophageal obstruction leads to copious secretions requiring frequent suctioning, and an inability to feed. Inability to pass the nasogastric tube into the stomach indicates oesophageal atresia.
- Obstruction in the proximal bowel above the ampulla of Vater results in non-bilious vomiting.
- Proximal bowel obstruction below the ampulla of Vater results in bilious vomiting with possibly some upper abdominal distension. Bilious (green) vomiting should always be taken seriously and is pathognomonic of gastrointestinal obstruction.
- Ileal, colonic and anal obstructions lead first to abdominal distension and subsequently to bilious vomiting. Dehydration secondary to third-space losses are larger the more distal the obstruction. Distal obstructions will present with failure to pass meconium (94% of newborns weighing more than 2500 g will pass stool in the first 24 hours and 99.8% will pass stool by 48 hours), although this is not invariable.

Radiological features Chest X-ray in oesophageal atresia may show a dilated, air-filled structure in the upper mediastinum indicating the proximal pouch. Proximal small bowel obstruction is indicated by a small number of dilated loops in the abdomen. Distal obstruction is suggested by multiple dilated bowel loops with air–fluid levels within them on upright or decubitus films. Radiologically it is impossible to tell the difference between large and small bowel on plain films in the neonate as the haustral folds are not well developed in the colon. Hence with a clinical and radiological distal bowel obstruction a lower gastrointestinal contrast study should be done to characterize the colon (microcolon, colonic plugs or transition zone, i.e. Hirschsprung's disease). Water-soluble contrast agents are normally used to minimize the risk associated with perforation.

PROXIMAL OBSTRUCTION

Oesophageal atresia

Clinical features Polyhydramnios is likely to be found, especially in pure oesophageal atresia. Postnatally, presenting features are a mucousy baby with apnoea and bradycardia, and an inability to pass a nasogestric tube into the stomach. Often there are associated anomalies such as VACTERL (Vertebral, Anorectal, Cardiac, Tracheo-oEsophageal, Renal, Limb) (see also p. 110).

Radiological appearance A chest and abdominal X-ray is required. A radio-opaque nasogastric tube will not pass into the stomach. Injection of air into the nasogastric tube at the same time as the chest/abdomen X-ray may delineate the size of the pouch and obviate a proximal pouch study with contrast. Gas within the bowel indicates a distal tracheo-oesophageal fistula (TOF): look for concomitant bowel distension, i.e. bowel obstruction, especially duodenal atresia. A gasless abdomen suggests absence of distal TOF and long gap oesophageal atresia. A proximal oesophageal 'pouchogram' can delineate the pouch size and the presence of proximal TOF, but there is a risk of aspiration if too much contrast is used.

Figure 4.1 shows a neonate with oesophageal atresia, as evidenced by the nasogastric tube which has turned on itself in a distended upper oesophagus. There is gas in the stomach, confirming a distal tracheo-oesophageal fistula. The infant was found to have oesophageal atresia and a tracheo-oesophageal fistula between the lower oesophagus and the trachea. This film is inadequate, however, as the full abdomen is not seen. On the one chest and abdominal film one should also look at the spine and number of ribs as part of the VACTERL syndrome.

Figure 4.2 shows anteroposterior (AP) and lateral views of the chest of a neonate with oesophageal atresia. Note the nasogastric tube in the air-filled upper oesophagus with a gasless abdomen, which characterizes oesophageal atresia without tracheo-oesophageal fistula. Sometimes if there is a small distal TOF it will take 24 hours for the air to reach the abdomen. Oesophageal atresia *without* a distal TOF often requires a delay to the initial repair, as the gap is too large and will need a gastrostomy initially.

Figure 4.3 demonstrates a proximal and distal TOF in a premature neonate. An upper gastrointestinal study has been performed and a large amount of contrast has passed into the tracheobronchial tree. There is air within the abdominal hollow viscera (i.e. distal TOF). The spine is normal. The contrast is water-soluble, but nonetheless is irritant to the airway, although it does not result in the toxic reactions seen with older contrast materials.

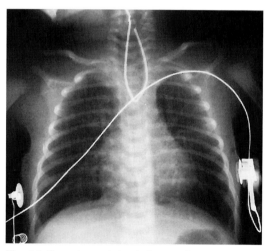

Fig. 4.1 Oesophageal atresia (see text).

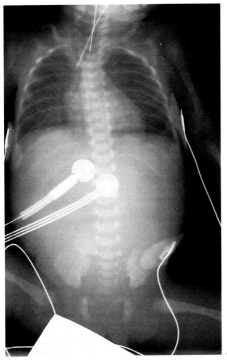

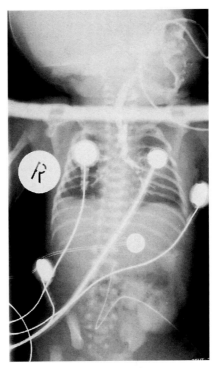

Fig. 4.3 Proximal and distal TOF in a premature neonate (see text).

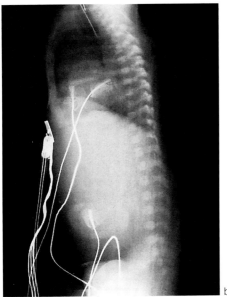

Fig. 4.2 Oesophageal atresia: (a) AP view; (b) lateral view.

The premature neonate shown in Figure 4.4 required vigorous resuscitation after birth. An AP film shows free air – there is air visible in the left and right side of the upper abdomen adjacent to the liver and spleen. If not looked for this can be missed on supine films. The lateral shoot-through confirms the presence of free air.

H-type tracheo-oesophageal fistula

Clinical features The H-type tracheo-oesophageal fistula does not cause a bowel obstruction but does cause recurrent pneumonia resulting from feeding-associated respiratory distress. These fistulas present later than oesophageal atresia and sometimes present only with stridor. The differential diagnosis includes seizure manifestations, apnoea syndromes and swallowing discoordination.

Radiographic appearance A prone lateral pull-back oesophagogram is required, and the procedure must be attended by both radiologists and clinicians. A normal study does not rule out an H-type TOF. Great care must be taken in performing this study as aspiration of contrast can lead to compromise of the respiratory status of the neonate. Figure 4.5 shows the relationship between the oesophagus and the trachea with an H-type fistula.

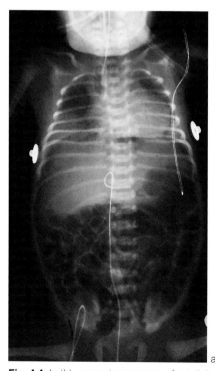

a

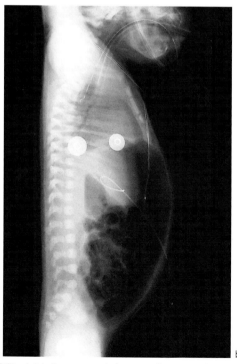

b

Fig. 4.4 In this premature neonate, free air is visible on the AP film (a) in the upper abdomen adjacent to the liver and spleen. Its presence was confirmed by the lateral shoot-through (b).

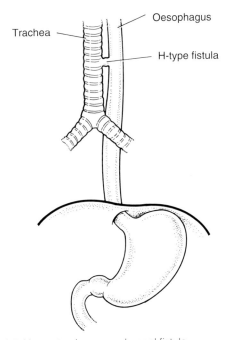

Oesophagus

Trachea

H-type fistula

Fig. 4.5 H-type tracheo-oesophageal fistula.

Figure 4.6 shows two films from a prone pull-back oesophagogram. The neonate is in the prone position with a nasogastric tube in the mid oesophagus. Contrast is injected as the tube is pulled back into the upper oesophagus. Contrast first outlines the oesophagus and then outlines the trachea in the same region, confirming the presence of a tracheo-oesophageal fistula. Overzealous injection of the oesophagus may lead to aspiration via the larynx and result in a falsely positive study. The oesophagus and trachea more distally were normal. Figure 4.7 shows an upper gastrointestinal study showing the 'kissing' of the trachea and oesophagus at the fistula site.

Rigid bronchoscopy in experienced hands is also sensitive in diagnosing both H-type tracheo-oesophageal fistula and proximal TOF with oesophageal atresia.

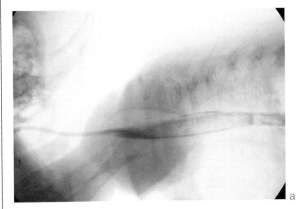
a

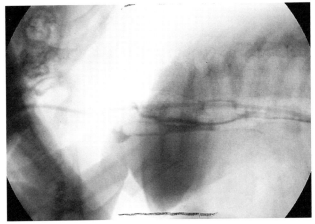
b

Fig. 4.6 Prone pull-back oesophagogram in a neonate with H-type TOF. Contrast outlines (a) the oesophagus and then (b) the trachea in the same region.

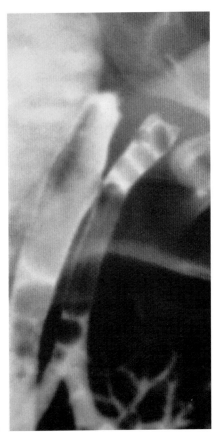

Fig. 4.7 H-type TOF: 'kissing' of trachea and oesophagus at fistula site.

Pyloric stenosis

Clinical features Postnatal onset of non-bilious vomiting which progressively worsens is indicative of pyloric stenosis. In full-term neonates the typical presentation is late (6 weeks of age), associated with an 'olive-sized mass'.

Radiological appearance Ultrasonography or an upper gastrointestinal X-ray series will demonstrate the anomaly. Ultrasound is the investigation of choice. Figure 4.8 shows an ultrasound image of pyloric stenosis. Note the elongated and thickened pylorus. Unfortunately, 'normal' size corrected standards are not yet available for preterm neonates, and even for full-term neonates are variable (Odbole et al 1996). Figure 4.9 shows an upper GI series on a neonate with recurrent non-bilious vomiting. There is a large amount of contrast in the stomach but little in the duodenum, with a long, narrow pylorus which is almost string-like, indicating pyloric stenosis (see arrow).

Pyloric atresia

Clinical features Polyhydramnios is found antenatally. Postnatally, non-bilious vomiting occurs in the first 24 hours of life with upper abdominal distension.

Radiological appearance Obstruction at the gastric outlet is visible on plain radiographs especially after injection of air through the nasogastric tube.

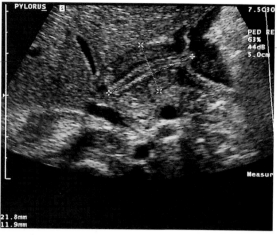

Fig. 4.8 Pyloric stenosis: ultrasound scan.

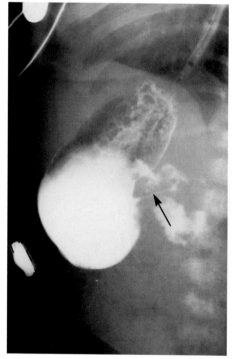

Fig. 4.9 Pyloric stenosis: upper GI series.

Duodenal atresia

Duodenal atresia is the most common cause of congenital duodenal obstruction.

Clinical features Signs are polyhydramnios antenatally and bilious vomiting postnatally. The condition is often associated with Down's syndrome.

Radiological appearance Duodenal atresia is usually not seen on antenatal ultrasound scans prior to 24 weeks gestational age. The 'double bubble' sign (Fig. 4.10) is a simultaneous distension of the stomach and first part of the duodenum; continuity between stomach and duodenum must be demonstrated. Polyhydramnios is invariably present.

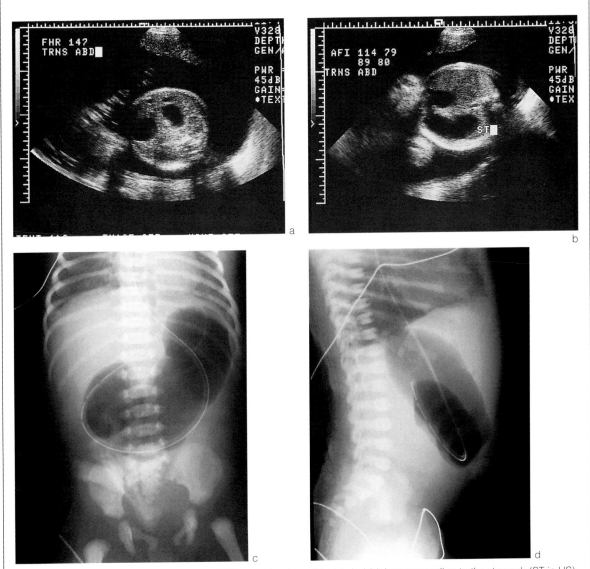

Fig. 4.10 Two images (a, b) from a prenatal US scan showing a 'double bubble' corresponding to the stomach (ST in US) and dilated duodenum. The fetal anatomy was otherwise unremarkable. There was associated polyhydramnios. Frontal and lateral films (c, d) taken postnatally show a dilated gas-filled stomach and proximal duodenum in an otherwise gasless abdomen. Air was injected into the stomach just prior to the plain films. The diagnosis of duodenal atresia was confirmed at surgery.

Duodenal stenosis

Clinical features Duodenal stenosis is characterized by bilious vomiting, which may present later than in duodenal atresia.

Radiological appearance Plain radiography shows the 'double bubble' with distal bowel gas (which rules out duodenal atresia) but does not rule out the urgent diagnosis of a malrotation with midgut volvulus; an upper GI study should be performed without delay (Figs. 4.11, 4.12).

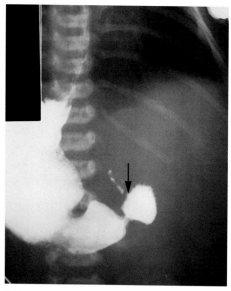

Fig. 4.11 Upper GI study demonstrating a stenosis of the duodenum just after the duodenal bulb (arrow).

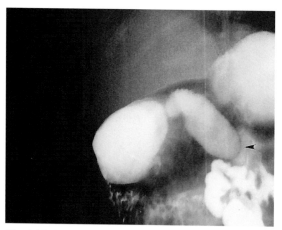

Fig. 4.12 A duodenal web is shown (arrow) in the second part of the duodenum.

Malrotation, volvulus

Clinical features Malrotation and volvulus often present as a sudden onset of bilious vomiting shortly after birth or in the first few months of life. Proximal obstruction is secondary to the midgut volvulus or Ladd's bands. Urgent diagnosis is needed to avoid catastrophic ischaemic injury to the midgut. Once diagnosed, Ladd's procedure for malrotation should proceed promptly.

Radiological appearance An upright abdominal X-ray in a newborn with bilious vomiting (Fig. 4.13a) shows the typical 'double bubble' sign but with distal bowel gas (hence ruling out duodenal atresia). The nasogastric tube is not far enough into the stomach to adequately decompress the obstruction. This X-ray could be seen in either duodenal stenosis or malrotation. An urgent upper GI study in the same neonate (Fig. 4.13b) shows a dilated (suggesting more chronic obstruction) first, second and part of third part of the duodenum. Contrast passes distally into less dilated bowel. This was radiologically interpreted to be duodenal stenosis. At the time of surgery the bowel was malrotated with a volvulus but was viable. Definite radiological differentiation between malrotation and duodenal stenosis may be difficult; if there is doubt, urgent surgery should be performed.

Figure 4.14 shows a single film from an upper GI series in a neonate with persistent vomiting, gas in the stomach and an otherwise gasless abdomen. There is obstruction at the second part of the duodenum. Surgery showed this was due to Ladd's bands associated with malrotation. From the film shown, duodenal atresia is impossible to rule out, as the contrast comes to a sudden and complete stop.

The radiological study of choice in malrotation is an upper GI series as it looks directly at the duodenal configuration (the duodenal C-loop of normal rotation). The barium enema looks only at the caecal position, which is often located in the right upper quadrant in normal neonates and therefore is not diagnostic of malrotation.

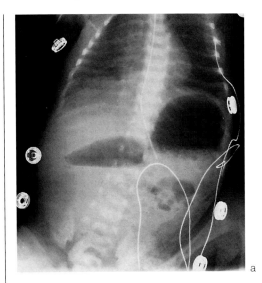

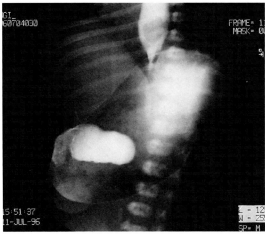

Fig. 4.14 Single film from an upper GI series in a neonate with persistent vomiting. Obstruction at the second part of the duodenum was shown at operation to be due to malrotation; duodenal atresia cannot be ruled out from this film.

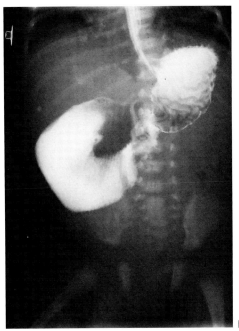

Fig. 4.13 Malrotation. An upright abdominal X-ray (a) shows the typical 'double bubble' sign but the distal bowel gas rules out duodenal atresia. (b) upper GI study in the same neonate (see text).

Jejunal atresia

Clinical features Bilious vomiting in the newborn period occurs in jejunal atresia. These infants may have severe electrolyte disorders secondary to vomiting.

Radiological appearance Figure 4.15 shows the classic features of jejunal atresia with the 'triple bubble' sign.

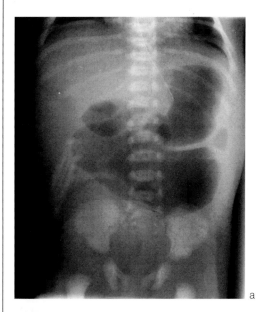

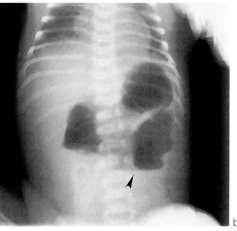

Fig. 4.15 Jejunal atresia. (a) Three air bubbles can be seen in an otherwise gasless abdomen: these bubbles represent air in the stomach (1), duodenal cap (2) and distal duodenum and proximal jejunum (3). The upright film (b) shows air fluid levels in the proximal jejunum (arrow).

DISTAL OBSTRUCTION

Ileal atresia

Clinical features Ileal atresia gives rise to abdominal distension, with bilious vomiting and palpable bowel loops.

Radiological appearance Multiple distended bowel loops are seen on X-ray; a contrast enema reveals a small (microcolon) large bowel. Figure 4.16 is a series of films of a neonate with atresia of the ileum. The last two films, from an upper GI study (UGI), were not necessary, as size discrepancy between the microcolon and distal ileum and the dilated non-opacified small bowel loops define the level of obstruction in the distal small bowel. An UGI series is not required and only delays definitive treatment, as one must wait for the colonic contrast material to exit the bowel before performing the UGI.

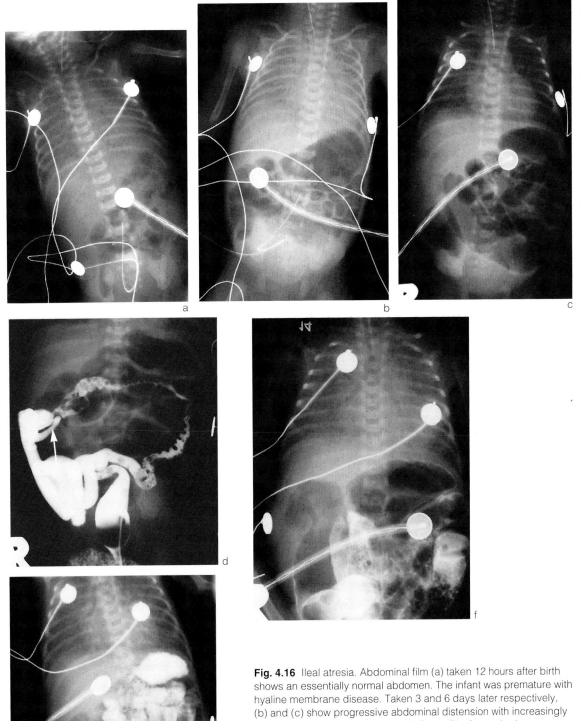

Fig. 4.16 Ileal atresia. Abdominal film (a) taken 12 hours after birth shows an essentially normal abdomen. The infant was premature with hyaline membrane disease. Taken 3 and 6 days later respectively, (b) and (c) show progressive abdominal distension with increasingly severely dilated loops of bowel. (d) Single film from a barium enema: the large bowel is small (microcolon) but otherwise normal. The caecum is in the right upper quadrant as shown by the appendix (arrow). Several loops of distal ileum are opacified and are of normal calibre. Two films (e, f) from an upper GI series show a normal upper jejunum with multiple distended loops of mid small bowel. Surgery confirmed ileal atresia.

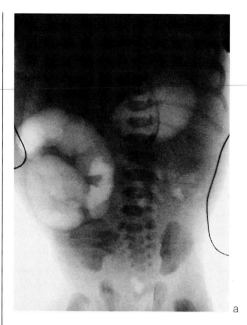

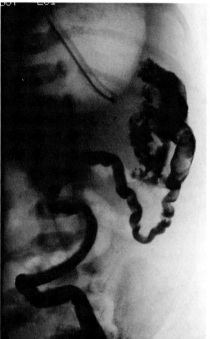

Meconium ileus

Clinical features Meconium ileus is characterized by abdominal distension, bilious vomiting and a 'doughy' abdomen (complicated meconium ileus).

Radiological appearance Multiple distended bowel loops are visible on X-ray. A contrast enema shows microcolon and thick meconium in the terminal ileum (Fig. 4.17). Investigate for cystic fibrosis.

The differential diagnosis of calcification on the abdominal X-ray in a neonate includes complicated meconium ileus, congenital infections (CMV) and adrenal haemorrhage. Delayed calcification may be seen in the mesenteric vessels after catheterization.

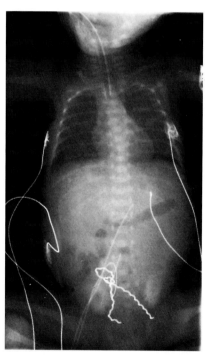

Fig. 4.17 Reversed image of a neonate with a distended abdomen demonstrates (a) a dominant dilated loop in the right side of the abdomen and some air in the stomach. (b) Microcolon seen in meconium ileus, with iatrogenic perforation with water-soluble contrast agent at the region of the splenic flexure.

Fig. 4.18 Single AP view of the chest and abdomen of a premature infant with hyaline membrane disease. Note the extensive abdominal calcifications as a result of perforation in utero and meconium spill (see right side of the spine and over the liver). There were no abdominal problems.

Meconium peritonitis

In complicated meconium ileus (antenatal perforation) there may be a soft tissue effect evident with or without intraabdominal calcification. Antenatal perforation is a cause of abdominal calcifications (Figs 4.18–4.20).

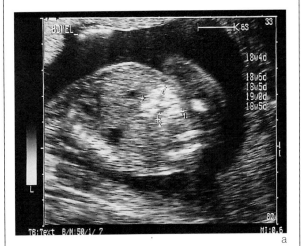

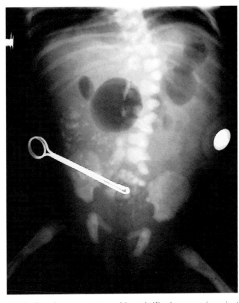

Fig. 4.20 Another neonate with calcified meconium in the abdomen (see right suprailiac area). This infant also had an imperforate anus, duodenal stenosis and spinal abnormalities.

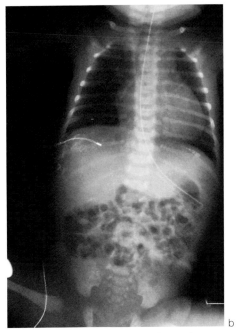

Fig. 4.19 Antenatal ultrasound scan (a) reveals intra-abdominal calcification in the fetus at 18 weeks gestation. Abdominal X-ray (b) in the same infant postnatally shows normal gas pattern but bilateral upper abdominal calcifications (see underneath both diaphragms). The child was asymptomatic in the neonatal period.

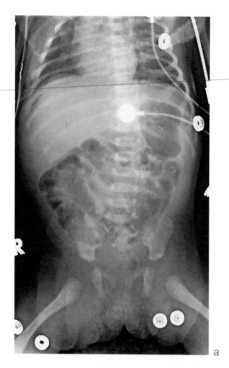

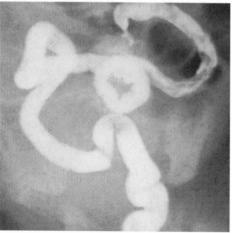

Fig. 4.21 Plain supine abdominal X-ray (a) demonstrates a distal bowel obstruction. Contrast enema (b) shows the microcolon ending blindly at the transverse colon. Colonic atresia was surgically corrected in this patient with a right hemicolectomy and a ileocolonic anastomosis.

Colonic obstruction

Clinical features Colonic obstruction presents with abdominal distension, bilious vomiting (later), palpable bowel loops and failure to pass meconium in first 24–48 hours.

Radiological appearance

- *Colonic atresia*: Figure 4.21.
- *Small left colon syndrome*: This distal obstruction is so named because of the appearance of the left colon on contrast enema. It is associated with maternal diabetes. This mimics a longer segment of colon in Hirschsprung's disease.
- *Meconium plug syndrome*: A contrast enema reveals multiple meconium plugs within the colon. This study is not only diagnostic but also therapeutic, as the neonate often passes the plugs after the study. The newborn shown in Figure 4.22 first passed a white plug and then continued to decompress after this study.

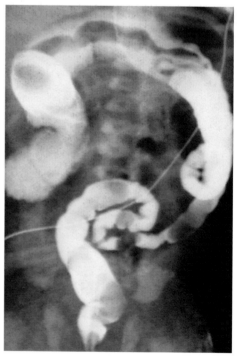

Fig. 4.22 Meconium plug syndrome.

Hirschsprung's disease

Clinical features Hirschsprung's disease is suggested by failure to pass meconium or stool (not invariable), abdominal distension and feeding intolerance with or without vomiting.

Radiological appearance A plain abdominal radiograph shows distended bowel loops and absence of rectal gas. (Fig. 4.23). A contrast enema demonstrates the transition zone (Figs 4.24, 4.25).

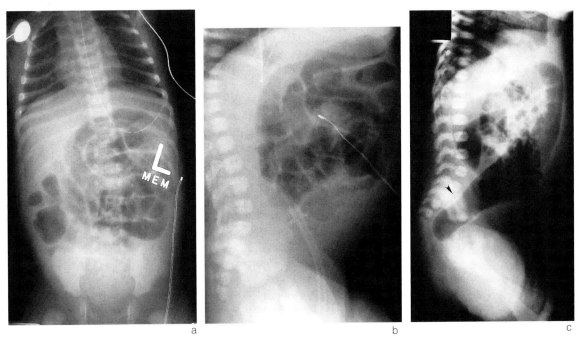

a   b   c

Fig. 4.23 (a,b) AP and lateral abdominal X-rays show distended loops of bowel and absence of gas in the lower abdomen and pelvis. (c) This plain lateral shoot-through suggests the transition zone (arrow). The lower sigmoid colon and rectum is smaller (aganglionic) then the dilated upper sigmoid colon.

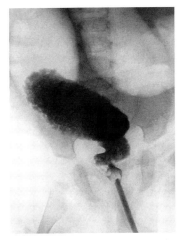

Fig. 4.24 The AP film of this contrast enema in an older infant demonstrates a small non-distended rectum with a dilated sigmoid colon (normally ganglionated) filled with gas. The contrast enema investigation of this child as a symptomatic neonate was normal and did not demonstrate a calibre difference in the lower colon.

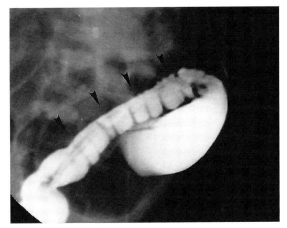

Fig. 4.25 The AP film of a contrast enema shows a longer segment (arrows) of Hirschsprung's disease with a transition zone in the upper sigmoid colon.

Figure 4.26 shows two films from a contrast enema in a patient who presented with a bowel obstruction. The plain film showed multiple loops of dilated bowel. Contrast enema showed a colon of normal calibre, but spiculation of the bowel was noted. This feature is suggestive of Hirschsprung's disease and is secondary to the spasm in the aganglionic bowel. Dilated, air-filled loops of small bowel were noted. Contrast fills the whole colon without observed peristalsis, again suggesting Hirschsprung's disease. The normal calibre of colon rules out not only large bowel obstruction but also distal small bowel atresia in which one would normally see a microcolon. This was later shown to be total-colon Hirschsprung's disease with extension of the aganglionosis 33 cm up the ileum. The colon can look normal on contrast examination with Hirschsprung's disease.

The patient in Figure 4.27 also had total-colon Hirschsprung's disease but showed a microcolon on contrast enema. The 5-week-old infant with diarrhoea since birth seen in Figure 4.28 presented with septic shock and a distended abdomen. The initial film showed dilated loops of bowel with stool present. Subsequent views of the abdomen after transport to a paediatric intensive care unit showed free air. This infant had total-colon Hirschsprung's disease with severe enterocolitis.

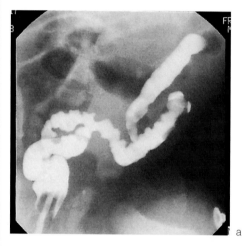

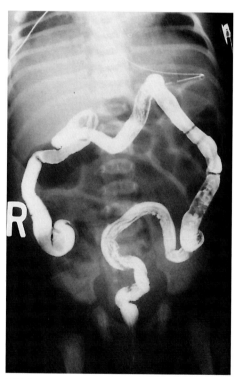

Fig. 4.27 Microcolon in a patient with total-colon Hirschsprung's disease.

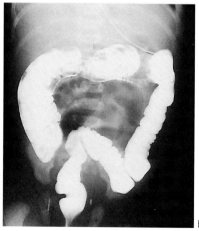

Fig. 4.26 (a,b) Two films from a contrast enema on a patient with bowel obstruction (see text).

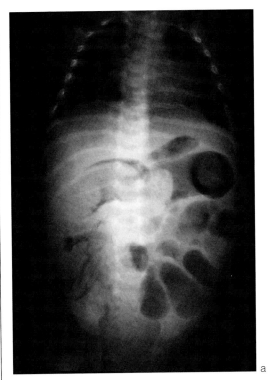

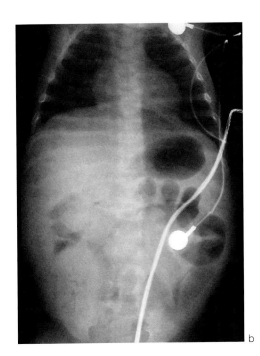

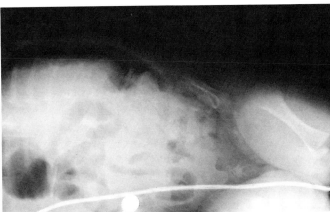

Fig. 4.28 Total-colon Hirschsprung's disease with severe enterocolitis in a 5-week-old infant with diarrhoea since birth. The initial film (a) shows dilated loops of bowel with stool present. Subsequent AP and lateral decubitus views (b,c) show free air.

Anal atresia: imperforate anus

Clinical features Absence or malposition of the anus may occur, with a distended abdomen. Male infants are likely to have a complete bowel obstruction and may pass meconium in the urine or to a perineal fistula. Females most commonly have a fistula to the vestibule of the introitus (posterior fourchette) and often pass meconium from this area. Look for other anomalies (i.e. VACTERL, p. 64).

Radiological appearance A prone lateral shoot-through demonstrates the level of the end of the bowel; an anteroposterior film may show an associated sacral anomaly. A distal contrast study in the cloacal variant of imperforate anus shows bifid uterus and the end of bowel to the cloaca.

Figure 4.29 shows an AP film demonstrating a distal bowel obstruction, and a prone lateral shoot-through of the pelvis with a marker on the anal area to define the distance between the end of the bowel and the skin. In this case the distance is long and the neonate required a colostomy. This film should be done when the neonate (and hence the bowel) is distended. The patient should be placed prone for 4–6 hours prior to this prone X-ray. It can be misleading if there is meconium at the end of the bowel.

Figure 4.30 shows a patient with a low imperforate anus. The sacral anomaly (scimitar sacrum) should always be looked for in imperforate anus. The ultrasound scan shows the usefulness of spinal ultrasonography in the neonate: a tethered cord is clearly seen with the cord ending at the L5–S1 level. This neonate also had a presacral teratoma in addition to the sacral anomaly and the imperforate anus (Currarino triad).

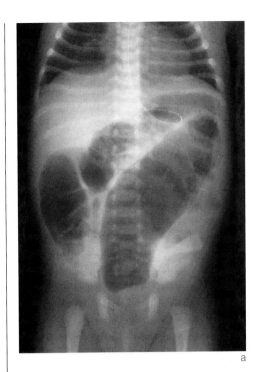

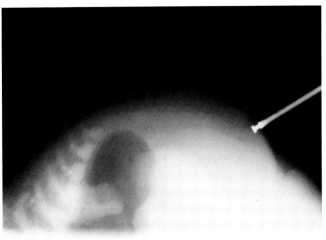

Fig. 4.29 Anal atresia. (a) AP film demonstrating distal bowel obstruction; (b) prone lateral shoot-through with a marker on the anal area to define the distance between the end of the bowel and the skin.

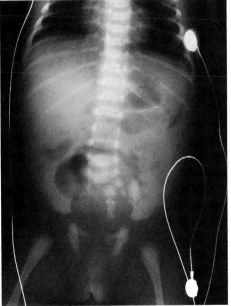

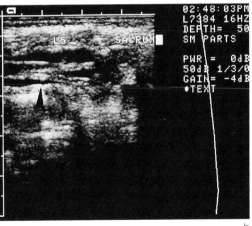

Fig. 4.30 Low imperforate anus. (a) Sacral anomaly (scimitar sacrum); (b) ultrasound scan showing tethered cord ending at the L5–S1 level (arrow).

NECROTIZING ENTEROCOLITIS

Clinical features

Necrotizing enterocolitis (NEC) is most common in premature and/or hypoxic babies who exhibit a combination of apnoea, bradycardia, temperature instability, intolerance to feeds (residuals, bilious and/or bloody aspirates or vomiting), respiratory failure, passage of gross or occult blood per rectum with variable abdominal findings. The role of infection is controversial, although 'epidemics' of necrotizing enterocolitis do occur, and secondary infections with septicaemia are common. The abdomen often becomes distended and tender, and may show focal cellulitis.

Radiological appearance

Typical features are pneumatosis intestinalis (the air pattern may be linear or 'bubbly'), air in the portal venous system, and free air (Figs 4.31–4.34). In the acute phase of NEC abdominal X-rays should be repeated every 6–8 hours or if there is a clinical change to suggest perforation. Late contrast radiographs may demonstrate strictures (Fig. 4.35).

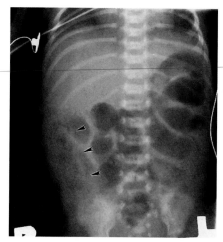

Fig. 4.31 Necrotizing enterocolitis. Abdominal view of a neonate with multiple distended loops of bowel. There is also a 'bubbly' pattern of air within the bowel wall (pneumatosis intestinalis) noted principally in the right colon (arrows).

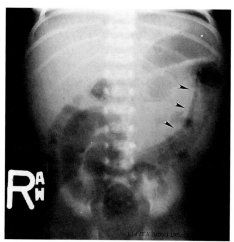

Fig. 4.32 In a second neonate with NEC the pneumatosis intestinalis is principally linear as seen in the left colon (arrows).

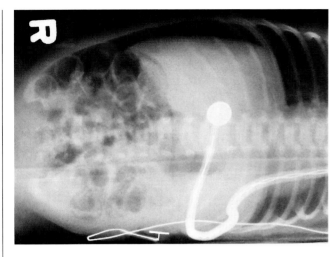

Fig. 4.33 A lateral decubitus film shows another neonate with NEC who has perforated and developed pneumoperitoneum.

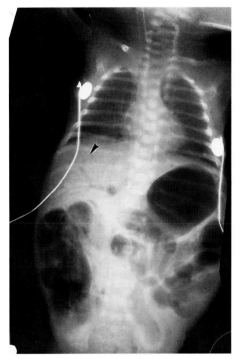

Fig. 4.34 An AP abdominal film in a neonate with NEC with air in the portal venous system (arrow).

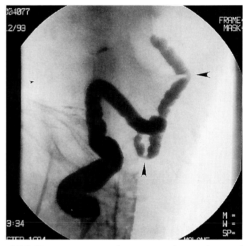

Fig. 4.35 Contrast enema shows two strictures (arrows) of the left colon in a neonate who had NEC. These were resected at the same time as the closure of the ileostomy.

HEPATIC LESIONS

Neonates with enlarging livers are most likely to have secondary spread from stage IVS neuroblastoma or nephroblastoma. Haemangiomas are the most common form of primary benign liver tumours and normally regress, but can lead to platelet sequestration (Kasabach–Merritt syndrome) and/or cardiac failure. Primary malignant liver tumours in the neonate are very rare. A typical radiologic appearance of such tumours is shown in Figure 4.36, which illustrates a case of haemangioendothelioma, presenting in cardiac failure.

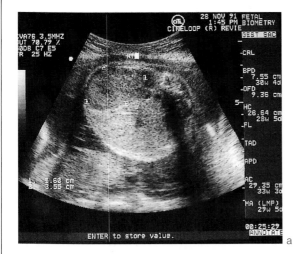

a

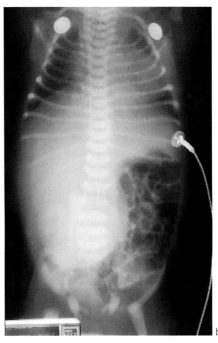

b

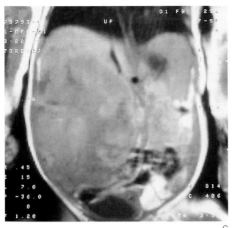

c

Fig. 4.36 An antenatal ultrasound scan (a) shows the mass in the upper abdomen. Fetal hydrops at 34 weeks gestation led to delivery by caesarean section. Plain abdominal X-ray (b) demonstrates the massive nature of the lesion. Magnetic resonance imaging (c) more fully delineates the anatomy. Right hepatic lobectomy was performed for heart failure with excellent outcome.

References

Beasley S W, Myers N A 1988 The diagnosis of congenital tracheoesophageal fistula. Journal of Pediatric Surgery 23: 415–417

Cohen M D, Schreiner R, Grosfeld J et al 1983 A new look at neonatal bowel-contrast studies with metrizamide. Journal of Pediatric Surgery 18: 442–448

Ghory M J, Sheldon C A 1985 Newborn surgical emergencies of the gastrointestinal tract. Surgical Clinics of North America 65: 1083–1098

Godbole P et al 1996 Ultrasound compared with clinical examination in infantile hypertrophic pyloric stenosis. Arch Dis Child 75: 335–337

Kasnak I, Senocak M, Hicsommez A et al 1997 The diagnosis and treatment of H-type tracheoesophageal fistulas. Journal of Pediatric Surgery 32(12): 1670–1674

Martin L W, Alexander F 1985 Esophageal atresia. Surgical Clinics of North America 65: 1099–1115

Powell D M, Othersen H B, Smith C D 1989 Malrotation of the intestines in children: the effect of age on presentation and therapy. Journal of Pediatric Surgery 24: 777–780

Simpson A J, Leonidas J C, Krasna I H et al 1972 Roentgen diagnosis of midgut malrotation: value of upper gastrointestinal radiographic study. Journal of Pediatric Surgery 7: 243–252

Walton M, Bass J, Soucy P 1995 Tethered cord with anorectal malformation, sacral anomalies, and presacral mass: an under reported association. European Journal of Pediatric Surgery 5: 59–62

Wheeler R 1994 Neonatal liver tumors. In: Freeman N V, Burge D M, Griffiths D M et al (eds) Surgery in the newborn, pp 533–537. Churchill Livingstone, Edinburgh

CHAPTER 5

The central nervous system

Cynthia Cupido
Haresh Kirpalani
John Mernagh

PRINCIPLES OF NEUROIMAGING

Choice of modality

Diseases of the germinal matrix

1. Ultrasonography (US) is the best modality for intraventricular haemorrhage, periventricular leukomalacia and posthaemorrhagic ventricular dilatation.
2. In addition US is repeatable, therefore it is uniquely useful.
3. If lesions of cystic periventricular leukomalacia are apparent on days 1–5 of life, suspect an intrauterine aetiology.

Trauma and asphyxia

1. Trauma requires computed tomography (CT) and possibly magnetic resonance imaging (MRI), as does asphyxia.
2. Ultrasonography illustrates only poorly the lesions of the posterior fossa – if these are suspected, obtain CT or MRI.
3. In prognosis for asphyxia and trauma, clinical evaluation and assessment are the most useful.

Complex problems associated with possible dysmorphism In complex developmental disorders detailed anatomical definition is required: MRI is essential.

Technical issues

MRI and CT Both MRI and CT pose special problems of monitoring, especially MRI where the infant is remote from access. Anaesthetic aid and/or advice may be needed for sedation and/or monitoring.

Ultrasound

1. Technically US power or brightness can alter the interpretation, but this depends on the observer.
2. Ensure the fontanelle window is large enough.
3. Repeated measurement of ventricular width at midcoronal points is the best method of following ventriculomegaly by US; it has less interobserver and intraobserver variability than other

measures (Levene 1981). At this site width does not vary with movement of the ultrasound beam. Other measures of vertical or oblique dimensions change considerably if the probe angle changes.

4. Related to the angle of insonation is a troublesome variation in Doppler flow velocity. This investigation is not therefore very useful clinically.

Guidelines for timing of 'routine' US screening in preterm infants

Early Ultrasound scans are needed in the following situations:

- Gestational age less than 32 weeks – a scan on day 1, repeated by day 7, will pick up most antenatal lesions and all new cases of intraventricular haemorrhage.
- Catastrophic event in preterm infant.

Late Ensure that follow-up US scans are completed by the time of discharge from the neonatal intensive care unit and/or at the corrected gestational age of 36 weeks. If the first scan is abnormal, repeat as required.

- If head growth is excessive or too little – scan weekly or more frequently. Normal head growth is about 1 mm per day.
- Use ultrasonography as a guide to surgical postoperative management of shunt insertion and its efficiency.
- Scan following acute severe hypoxaemia and recovery, at about 5–7 days for cystic lesions.

NEUROANATOMY

Figures 5.1 and 5.2 illustrate anatomy referred to in this chapter. Figure 5.1 shows two coronal views and two sagittal views through the brain, which can be directly compared with the US scans shown in Figure 5.2.

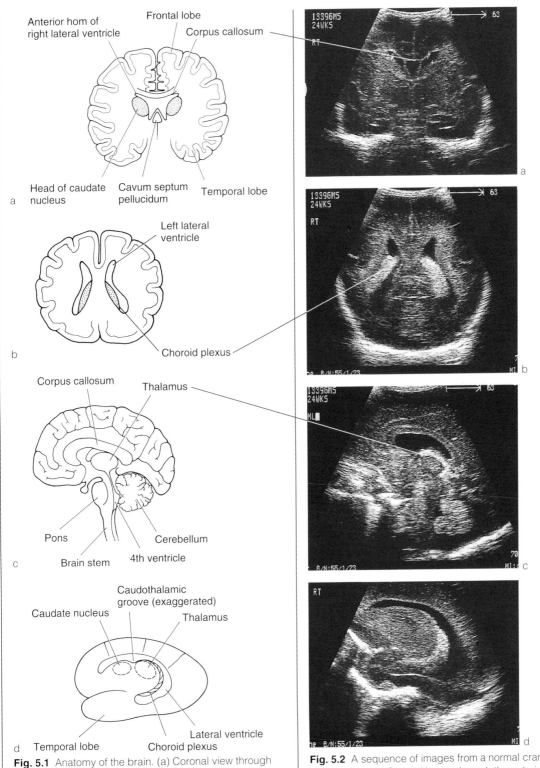

Fig. 5.1 Anatomy of the brain. (a) Coronal view through the anterior horns; (b) coronal view through the bodies of the lateral ventricles; (c) sagittal view through the midline; (d) sagittal view through the right lateral ventricle. These can be directly compared with the images in Fig. 5.2.

Fig. 5.2 A sequence of images from a normal cranial US examination. (a) Coronal image through the anterior horns; (b) coronal image through the bodies of the lateral ventricles; (c) sagittal image through the midline; (d) sagittal image through the right lateral ventricle.

Figure 5.3 shows the so-called 'homunculus' at the cortical level, and the associated corticospinal tracts that are impinged upon by penetrating grade 4 IVH and are affected by the process of cystic change in PVL.

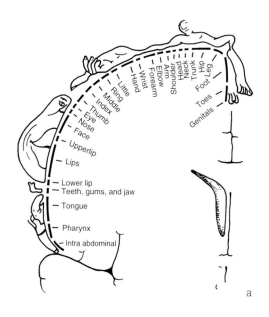

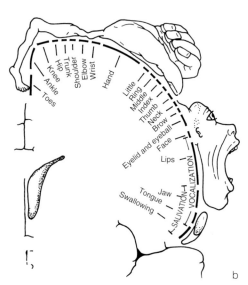

Fig. 5.3 Sensory (a) and motor (b) homunculus, drawn overlying a coronal section through the precentral gyrus. From Fig. 1.5 Chusid J G, in Correlative neuroanatomy and functional neurology, 18th edn, Los Altos, and Fig. 100 in 'Functional neuroanatomy' by Everett N V and Boedmer C W, Rieke WO. Philadelphia.

HAEMORRHAGIC AND ISCHAEMIC LESIONS RELATED TO THE GERMINAL MATRIX

There is a spectrum of haemorrhagic and ischaemic conditions from an initial haemorrhage through to cystic change and ventricular dilatation. Once a bleed has occurred, apart from its intrinsic effects there are other pathological changes. First, there is a decrease of underlying venous flow, which exacerbates the preterm pressure passive cerebral circulation; compensation for swings from low to high arterial blood pressure is absent, and subsequent ischaemia may develop. Secondly, there may be an obstruction to the flow of cerebrospinal fluid (CSF). The three conditions discussed below may have a similar aetiology, but the prognostic and therapeutic problems they pose are quite different.

Intraventricular haemorrhage

Definition and aetiology Intraventricular haemorrhage (IVH) is a frequent complication of prematurity between 24 weeks and 30 weeks of gestation. The subependymal germinal matrix, or choroid plexus, is a vascular structure found only in the preterm brain (Pape & Wigglesworth 1979). In preterm infants most IVH arises from this structure. Investigation of platelets and coagulation factors in most cases of preterm IVH are normal. Little evidence to date supports an important role in aetiology for abnormalities in platelets or coagulation factors. Other risk factors for IVH include asphyxia, respiratory distress syndrome and its complications (e.g. pneumothorax, respiratory acidosis), early hypotension and fluctuating cerebral blood flow velocity (as when infant and ventilator are out of synchrony).

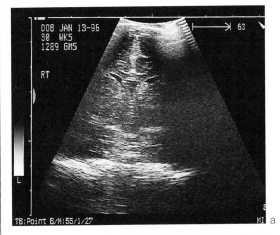

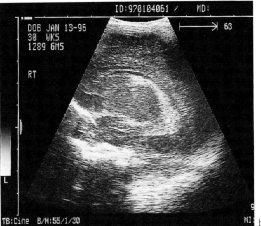

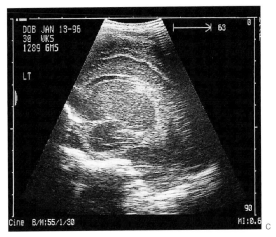

Fig. 5.4 Typical example of a right grade 1 and a left grade 2 IVH; (a) coronal (see crosses on image) and (b, c) sagittal images through the right and left lateral ventricles. Note the increased echogenicities in the subependymal regions in comparison with Fig. 5.2. The left grade 2 IVH is very subtle and can easily be mistaken for a grade 1 IVH.

Clinical features Intraventricular haemorrhage usually occurs in babies of less than 30 weeks gestational age unless severe illness supervenes. Since 80% of IVH have occurred by 72 hours after delivery, routine US scanning at the end of the first week in infants of gestational age less than 33 weeks will reveal virtually all cases of IVH.

The clinical picture varies by both degree of bleed and by anatomical location. The latter provides a classification into four grades. Small haemorrhages confined to the subependymal region (grade 1) or small IVH (grade 2) are not usually accompanied by clinical signs or sequelae. Only 'routine' US will pick up these lesions (Figs 5.4, 5.5). Follow-up shows no associated cerebral palsy or disability in grade 1 and 2 IVH. Nevertheless, posthaemorrhagic ventricular dilatation (PHVD) developing after a grade 2 IVH may have clinical significance.

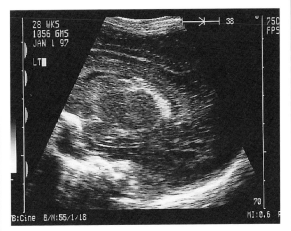

Fig. 5.5 Sagittal image of another neonate with a grade 2 IVH that is a little more obvious than in Fig. 5.4. Since the choroid plexus itself is echogenic, a small IVH may be called by some observers a 'full choroid plexus'.

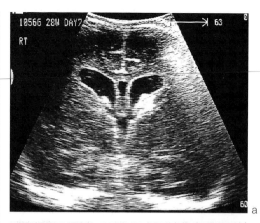

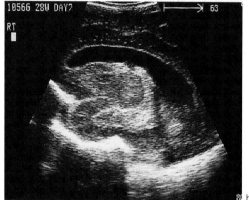

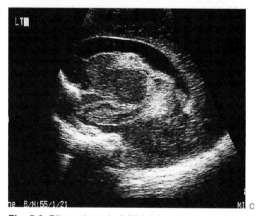

Fig. 5.6 Bilateral grade 3 IVH; (a) coronal and (b) right and left sagittal images. Note the enlargement of the lateral ventricles.

Rarely, large IVH with associated dilatation of the ventricular system (grade 3) is accompanied by hypotonia and seizures, shock and a drop in haemoglobin level. Grade 3 IVH has a 20–50% risk of PHVD and hydrocephalus (Fig. 5.6).

A grade 4 IVH involves injury to the brain's parenchyma (Fig. 5.7). The degree of the blood loss is variable; if large it may present in the same way as a large grade 3 haemorrhage, but the risk of seizure is higher with grade 4. Ultrasonographic follow-up of grade 3 and grade 4 IVH at least twice a week is needed to detect PHVD and the liquefaction of parenchymal lesions to porencephalic cysts.

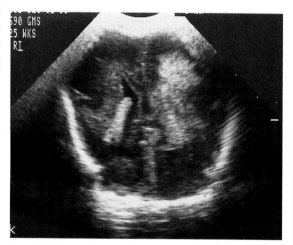

Fig. 5.7 Coronal image of a neonate with grade 4 IVH. Note the large intraparenchymal echogenicity just lateral to the left lateral ventricle.

Periventricular leukomalacia

Clinical features An injury to the periventricular white matter, periventricular leukomalacia (PVL) may result from an inadequate initial blood flow with later hyperaemia during the reperfusion phase following injury. This condition is most common in infants of 28–32 weeks gestational age. The frequency of cystic PVL is approximately 3% in infants with birthweights less than 1500 g. Periventricular leukomalacia is associated with antepartum haemorrhage and placental abruption; multiple pregnancy, particularly twin-twin transfusion, and death of one twin; prolonged rupture of the membranes and chorioamnionitis; hypocapnia during mechanical ventilation (e.g. overventilation); sepsis, hypotension and necrotizing enterocolitis. In mild cases, no cavitation occurs but gliosis forms a permanent scar. More severe cases have cavities – 'cystic PVL'. The position and extent of the cysts in part determine the prognosis. Since the white matter affects myelination of the corticospinal tract, the most medial fibres of which control movement in the legs, spastic diplegia is the most common neurological disability (see Fig. 5.3).

Radiological appearance

Classification of PVL by US findings The diagnosis is best made by US with a frequency of 7 MHz, 7.5 MHz or higher (Pidcock et al 1990, De Vries et al 1992). Initial periventricular echodensities are usually symmetrical with edges, and lesions still separable from the ventricle edge. Confirm that the echodensity is at least as dense as the choroid plexus, and confirm the echodensity in at least two views, e.g. coronal and sagittal.

Cyst evolution Cavitation or cyst formation takes 2–4 weeks after the initial cerebral insult and appears as echolucencies within a previous echodensity. Echolucencies are usually multiple, and separate from the ventricular system. In contrast, porencephalic cysts are usually single and communicate with the ventricular system. Cysts as small as 2 mm can be visualized.

Timing of the cerebral insult Since cyst formation usually takes at least 2 weeks, lesions can often be 'timed'. If cystic lesions are clearly seen within 7 days, then an antepartum cause is likely. A normal scan soon after birth followed by the appearance of echodensities, and then cyst formation in 2–4 weeks, indicates a postnatal cerebral insult.

Prognosis in PVL from imaging – site and timing

1. If lesions are present on day 1 suspect an intrauterine process. This implies a worse prognosis.
2. Some echodensities disappear within a week (transient echodensities or flares) and do not imply an increased risk of cerebral palsy.
3. Other echodensities persist for weeks (grade 1 PVL) and do represent an increased risk of cerebral palsy (around 20% if extensive).
4. Echolucencies restricted to the frontal area (grade 2 PVL) represent an only slightly increased risk of cerebral palsy.
5. Extensive echolucencies in the frontal and temporal areas (grade 3 PVL) have a high risk of cerebral palsy (60–80%), often with

mental retardation, visual impairment and epilepsy. Frontal cystic PVL may be difficult to distinguish from subependymal cyst formation (e.g. after a small grade 1 IVH) which has a good prognosis.

Figure 5.8 shows the progression of a grade 4 IVH over the course of a month.

Posthaemorrhagic ventricular dilatation

Posthaemorrhagic ventricular dilatation is a sequela to IVH grade 3, and was once thought to be a simple obstruction from the coagulated clot. It is likely to be more complex in reality, with some gliosis and fibrosis.

Definition and clinical significance One definition is both quantitative and reproducible, and will identify infants at 50% or greater risk of shunt dependence (i.e. placing of ventriculoperitoneal shunts and/or cerebral palsy). This is the presence of intraventricular haemorrhage on an early US scan, with:

- *either* a progressive increase in midcoronal ventricular width
- *or* a midcoronal ventricular width reaching 4 mm beyond the 97th percentile (Ventriculomegaly Trial Group 1990).

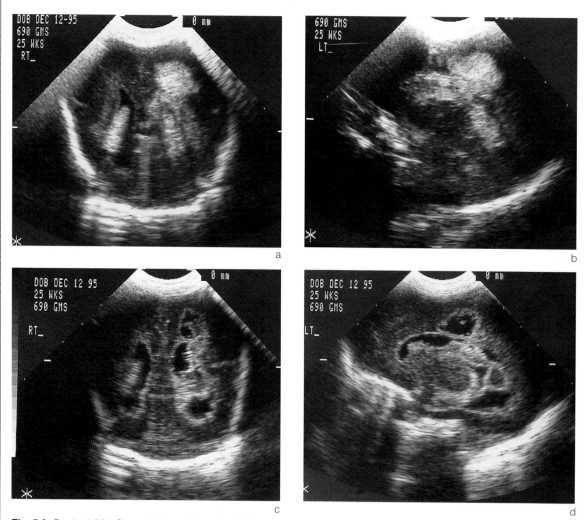

Fig. 5.8 Grade 4 IVH. Coronal (a) and left sagittal (b) images from the first examination performed a few days after birth in a neonate of 25 weeks gestation. Note the large area of increased echogenicity just lateral and superior to the left lateral ventricle. After 1 month these echogenicities have become cystic in nature (c, d). In the second scan thrombus is seen in the left lateral ventricle (d).

Treatment Most would attempt to delay surgery as spontaneous resolution may still occur (e.g. Fig. 5.9). Randomized evaluation of repeat lumbar puncture showed no benefit, but may serve to delay surgery (and thus potential infection) to a less critical juncture.

Radiological appearance Ventricular width measurements are most sensitive for first detecting enlargement, but not so useful in detecting further changes with very large ventricles, mainly because the ventricular system enlarges occipitally later on. Figures 5.9 and 5.10 are two series of US images from two neonates with PHVD.

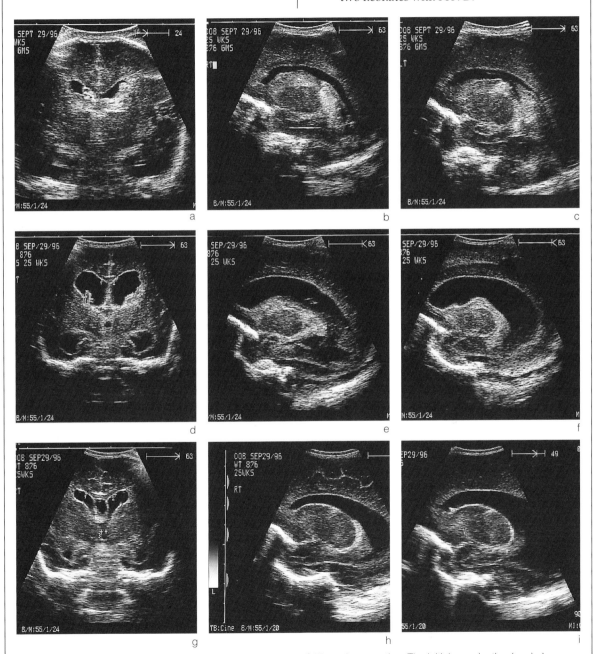

Fig. 5.9 Posthaemorrhagic ventricular dilatation in a neonate of 25 weeks gestation. The initial examination (a–c) shows bilateral grade 3 IVH, in both coronal (a) and left and right sagittal (b, c) views. One week later the lateral ventricles are significantly dilated (d–f). After another week there has been spontaneous decrease in the ventricular dilatation without active intervention (g–i).

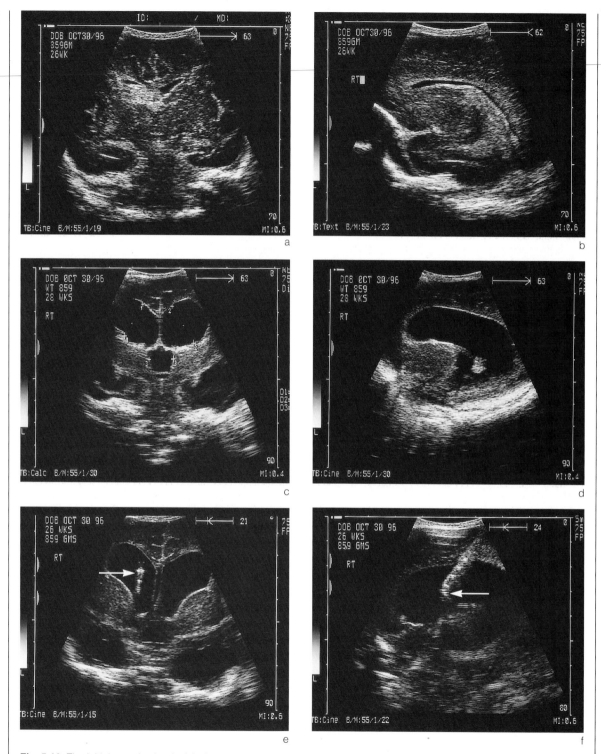

Fig. 5.10 The initial examination (a, b) of a second neonate of 25 weeks gestation shows a right grade 2 IVH. One week later there is severe ventricular dilatation (c, d). This did not resolve and required placement of a shunt (e, f). Arrows show the tip of the shunt.

CEREBRAL INFARCTION

Clinical features

Focal clonic seizures within 3 days of birth may be due to localized cerebral infarction. Usually, this is in the territory of the middle cerebral artery. The electroencephalogram (EEG) is usually asymmetrical. Some infants may have developed infarction before birth, by paradoxical embolism (through the foramen ovale) of placental thrombi. A particularly severe form is *hydrancephaly*, which is seen after an early in utero episode (Fig. 5.12).

Radiological appearance

Diagnosis is only suggested by US, and is best confirmed by CT at 48 hours. The CT scan shows parenchymal loss, with a porencephalic cyst or localized dilatation of one lateral ventricle. In the absence of general asphyxia the prognosis can be relatively good, with half of these babies showing no major disability and half with degrees of hemiplegia (Figs 5.11, 5.12). Treatment with anticoagulation remains controversial at this time, and expert haematological and neurological opinion should be sought.

HYPOXIC–ISCHAEMIC ENCEPHALOPATHY AND FULL-TERM BIRTH ASPHYXIA

Definition and clinical features

Fetal distress is followed by delivery of a white or blue infant with a persistently low Apgar score and/or low cord blood pH (< 7.0). After resuscitation the infants may have encephalopathy usually evident within 48 hours. This is usually graded as mild (grade 1), moderate (grade 2) or severe (grade 3) (Sarnat & Sarnat 1976). In moderate and severe cases, clinical and EEG seizures are common. Look for multiorgan injury, impaired circulation, myocardial ischaemia (ECG), and decreased renal and liver function. The prognosis is best indicated by clinical progress over time, including seizure presence, presence of sucking and responsiveness. Imaging will exclude neurological causes, malformations and prenatal lesions; EEG will document seizure and may assist prognosis – especially if masking drugs are present, or if the infant is paralysed to assist ventilation.

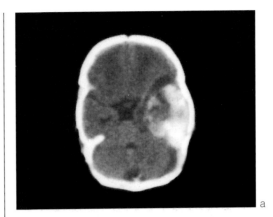
a

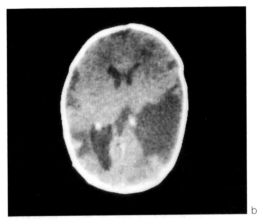
b

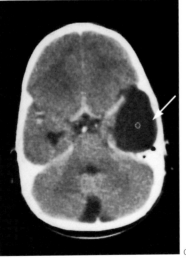
c

Fig. 5.11 Cerebral infarction: CT scans of a neonate who presented initially with a large intraparenchymal haemorrhage involving most of the left temporal lobe, as seen by the large bright area which represents fresh blood (a). Within a few weeks the blood has resolved (b) and after 1 year there is a large area of porencephaly involving the left temporal region (c) (arrow).

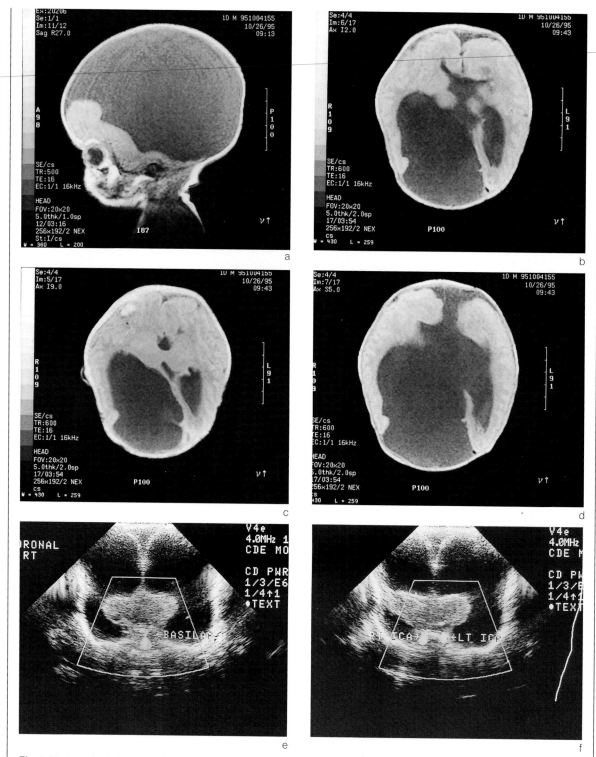

Fig. 5.12 A particularly severe form of cerebral infarction known as hydrancephaly, resulting from infarction of all the brain perfused by the internal carotid arteries. Films a–d show coronal and sagittal images from an MRI scan of a neonate showing severe destruction of brain parenchyma involving all the brain except that perfused by the posterior circulation. A scan using Doppler ultrasonography (e,f) showed flow in the carotid arteries and the basilar artery but no flow in the supraclinoid carotid arteries.

Radiological appearance

Ultrasounds may be 'subjectively' read as showing increased echodensity ('bright brain') in severe encephalopathy with cerebral oedema. Radiology is however only ancillary, and emphasis should be on the clinical and EEG picture. Very high-frequency US (10 MHz) demonstrates focal lesions early. A CT scan is helpful, but not in the first 24–48 hours (because of cerebral oedema), to show the extent of injury in the hemispheres with low attenuation areas. (Fig. 5.13). Magnetic resonance imaging may show the distribution of hypoxic–ischaemic encephalopathy (HIE), but not all infants with severe HIE have widespread early visible cortical damage. Lesions in the thalamus, basal ganglia and brain stem may be seen. Diffusion-weighted MRI looks promising for early visualization of the extent of damage. Follow-up imaging is useful in infants who remain neurologically abnormal after 1 week, as early signs of atrophy carry a poor prognosis. Unfortunately MRI is impractical in acute cases, where parental counselling may be required with a view to decision-making; emphasis should be on the clinical picture. Incidentally, brain death determination is not generally applicable in the newborn, though some have advocated Xenon flow studies.

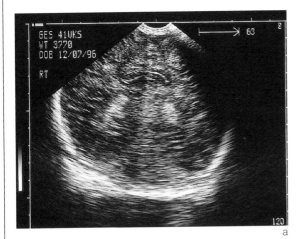
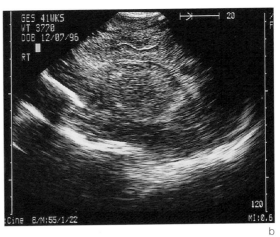

a

b

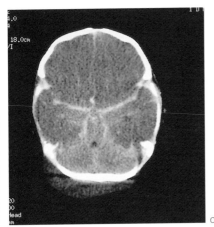
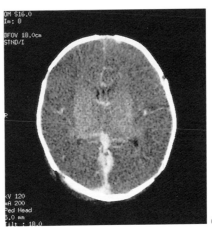

c

d

Fig. 5.13 Coronal (a) and sagittal (b) images from an US examination in a neonate suspected of suffering a hypoxic event; these images are essentially normal. The CT scans (c, d) show generalized decrease in the density of the cerebral hemispheres in relation to the cerebellum and basal ganglia.

CEREBRAL ATROPHY

The term 'cerebral atrophy' is used to denote a loss of brain tissue. It is generally not a clinical finding but is usually only noted on scanning; except in severe conditions of antenatal aetiology, usually developmental. There may be microcephaly. In preterm infants the appearance of atrophy by US may be of no clinical importance (Lui et al 1990).

Differential diagnosis

As well as the more common cerebrospinal fluid hydrocephalus, there is sometimes an 'external' hydrocephalus. Here transient enlargement of the subarachnoid space is seen, with head enlargement, but without evidence of subarachnoid haemorrhage. The prognosis is good. It is important to distinguish this from subdural effusion, posthaemorrhagic hydrocephalus and cerebral atrophy (Ment et al 1981):

- Measurements of head circumference over 2–3 weeks may be helpful: cerebral atrophy is not usually associated with excessive head growth, and hydrocephalus is. The clinical signs of hydrocephalus with vomiting, 'sunsetting', tense fontanelle, splayed sutures, etc., may also help (see below).
- In cerebral atrophy, ventricular dilatation is often irregular and slightly asymmetrical; in hydrocephalus, the lateral ventricles are usually ballooned.
- In pure atrophy, look for a widening of the interhemispheric and sylvian fissures.

Radiological appearance

Radiography simply shows large fluid spaces. Sometimes apparent 'ventricular dilatation' is due to cerebral atrophy rather than CSF pressure-driven hydrocephalus. In atrophy, the brain is too small for the skull and there is an increase in the subarachnoid space, fissures and ventricular system. With only a single examination, either by US or CT, it is difficult to distinguish atrophy from hydrocephalus. Figure 5.14 shows a single coronal image of a neonate with cerebral atrophy. Note the increased distance between the cerebral cortex and the inner border of the cranium. The sulci are still rounded, which is consistent with atrophy rather than a subdural haemorrhage in which the sulci would be flattened.

CONGENITAL HYDROCEPHALUS

Congenital hydrocephalus may be an isolated finding due to aqueduct stenosis, or it may be part of a more widespread disturbance of brain development such as:

1. the Arnold–Chiari malformation type 2 in which the infant has a lumbar meningomyelocele together with caudal dislocation of the medulla oblongata and cerebellar vermis
2. atresia of the foramen of Magendie leading to gross enlargement of the fourth ventricle into the cisterna magna with secondary atrophy of the cerebellar vermis: the Dandy–Walker malformation
3. that associated with encephalocele
4. that associated with an inherited metabolic disease, e.g. achondroplasia or mucopolysaccharidosis
5. craniofacial dysmorphisms, e.g. Alpert's or Crouzon's disease
6. congenital hydrocephalus from intrauterine infection (e.g. toxoplasmosis), intrauterine intracranial haemorrhage or neoplastic and vascular malformations.

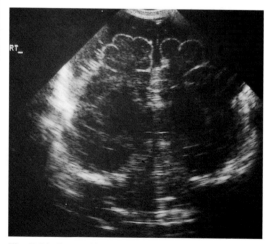

Fig. 5.14 Coronal image of a neonate with cerebral atrophy with a large space above the cortex.

Clinical features

The clinical features of CSF-driven hydrocephalus are excessive head enlargement or raised intracranial pressure. The head circumference is above the 97th centile, or 2 centile lines above the weight centile; or there is a rapid increase in head circumference exceeding the normal neonatal head growth of about 1 mm a day. Other signs may include a very broad or tense fontanelle, irritability, vomiting and abnormal eye movements with failure of upward gaze ('sunsetting').

Radiological appearance

Demonstrating anatomical dilatation of the ventricular system is not enough as the appearance may be due to atrophy. The distinction between atrophy and hydrocephalus is important as causes, prognosis and management are different (see above). Even a slight suspicion of hydrocephalus should prompt US investigation for ventricular width in the midcoronal view (reference values above). If in doubt, a repeat head circumference measurement and cranial US in a few days or a week is decisive. The US scan may indicate the cause, e.g. traces of blood clot, or calcification indicating old ventriculitis. Determine to what extent the third ventricle is dilated and compare this with the fourth ventricle (Fig. 5.15). In aqueduct obstruction, the fourth ventricle is not dilated, but if a large fourth ventricle or cyst can be seen, this suggests obstruction of the foramens of Magendie and Luschka. In suspected cerebral malformation in association with hydrocephalus, MRI will define the abnormality better; US is useful, together with repeated head circumference, in monitoring treatment.

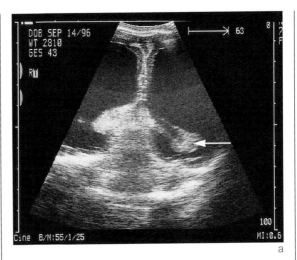

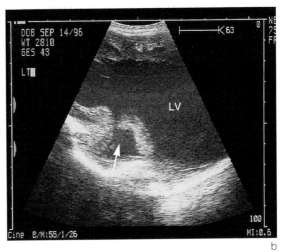

Fig. 5.15 Coronal (a) and sagittal (b) images from an US examination of a neonate with gross hydrocephalus. In this case the third ventricle was not enlarged (arrow in (b)), leading to the diagnosis of obstruction at the level of the foramen of Monro. (LV, lateral ventricle.)

AGENESIS OF THE CORPUS CALLOSUM

The corpus callosum allows nerve fibre communication between the left and the right hemispheres. Agenesis or hypoplasia is an important sign of brain malformation, and occurs in a number of conditions including inherited metabolic diseases.

Clinical features

Clinical clues to agenesis are hypertelorism, ocular abnormalities, cleft palate and malformations of the digits. However, not all infants with agenesis have neurological signs.

Radiological appearance

Ultrasonography shows absence of the characteristic double curve of the corpus callosum seen on the sagittal view, and the third ventricle may be higher than usual (Fig. 5.16). Lateral ventricles may appear slightly further apart than normal (Fig. 5.17) and may be slightly dilated. The finding of agenesis or hypoplasia of the corpus callosum should prompt a search for other clinical abnormalities, chromosome analysis and anatomical delineation by MRI.

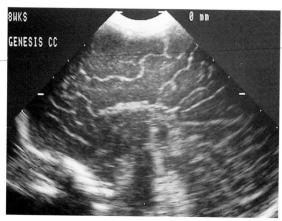

Fig. 5.16 Sagittal US image through the midline showing absence of the corpus callosum with a high third ventricle.

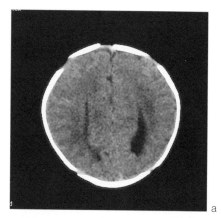

a

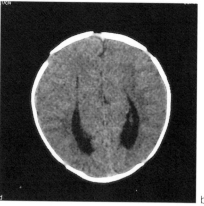

b

Fig. 5.17 Two CT images showing absence of the corpus callosum as noted by the lateral ventricles which appear slightly further apart and more parallel than normal.

NEURONAL MIGRATION DEFECTS

Neuronal multiplication before 20 weeks of gestation is followed by migration (e.g. from the germinal matrix) to different cortical layers. A generalized disturbance of migration results in an abnormal gyral pattern associated with severe neurological dysfunction. The disorders known as the lissencephalies (agyria) have no sulci visible, although the sylvian fissure is visible.

Clinical features

Constellations of abnormalities may be the clue to underlying cerebral problems. The Miller–Dieker syndrome includes lissencephaly, fetal polyhydramnios, prominent forehead, small jaw, bitemporal hollowing, mental retardation and infantile spasms. However, isolated lissencephaly can occur without dysmorphic features. Rarer syndromes may be present, e.g. the Walker–Warburg syndrome (absence of cerebral and cerebellar gyri, hydrocephalus, retinal dysplasia and encephalocele) or Zellweger's syndrome, a peroxisomal disorder. Periventricular heterotopias occur when a group of neurones have failed to migrate and remain in the periventricular region. These masses may protrude into the ventricular lumen and are visible on CT or MRI, but some are asymptomatic. Figure 5.18 is a film from a CT examination showing an extreme case of lissencephaly in which there are no sulci or gyri present.

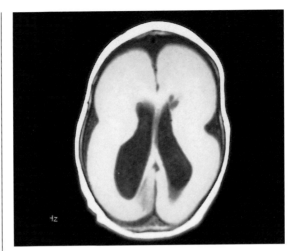

Fig. 5.18 Lissencephaly. No sulci or gyri are present on this CT scan.

HOLOPROSENCEPHALY

Holoprosencephaly is a spectrum of defects in midline cleavage of the embryonic forebrain. The mildest form is absence of the olfactory tracts and bulbs. The most severe form involves a proboscis and the 'cyclops' deformity (single eye).

Clinical features

Cyclops deformity is obvious. Suspect alobar holoprosencephaly clinically with hypertelorism, flat nose, absent philtrum; as part of trisomy 13 and 13q syndromes and trisomy 18 and 18p syndromes.

Radiological appearance

Ultrasonography characteristically reveals an undivided ventricular cavity in the anterosuperior brain. The temporal horns of the ventricular system are differentiated. There is an incomplete interhemispheric fissure anteriorly. Figures 5.19 and 5.20 are two examples of neonates with holoprosencephaly first seen with US. The first neonate is less severely affected; there is almost complete coalescence of the lateral ventricles, which still remain undivided in the midline. In the second neonate there is a single monoventricle. Incidental note is made of the small intraventricular haemorrhages seen in the first neonate.

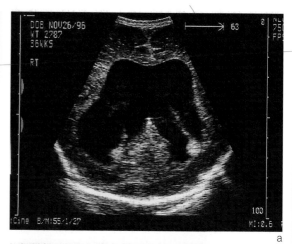

a

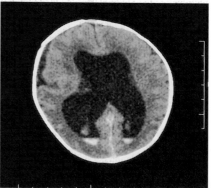

b

Fig. 5.19 Holoprosencephaly. There is almost complete fusion/coalescence of the lateral ventricles, which are undivided in the midline. Small IVH are visible.

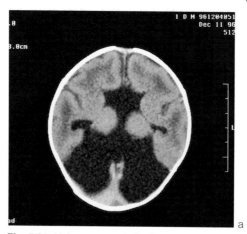

a

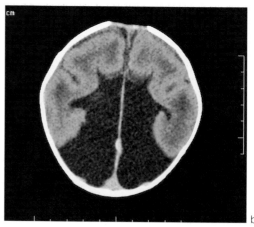

b

Fig. 5.20 Holoprosencephaly. A more severe case than that in Fig. 5.19, with a single ventricle.

TRAUMATIC INTRACRANIAL HAEMORRHAGE: SUBDURAL HAEMORRHAGE

Subdural haemorrhage includes:

1. tentorial 'tear' with haemorrhage from the straight sinus, transverse sinus or vein of Galen
2. falx laceration with rupture of the inferior sagittal sinus
3. rupture of superficial cerebral convexity veins.

Clinical features

The clinical history usually describes a full-term infant with a face or brow presentation in which the head is subjected to greater than normal deforming stresses. Alternatively, there has been a difficult forceps or vacuum extraction. The clinical picture varies with the extent and site of the trauma. Severe cases are in very poor condition at birth and require resuscitation, but fail to achieve normal consciousness and activity. Unilateral convexity haemorrhages may present with poor condition at birth, subsequent focal seizures and an asymmetrical pupillary reaction.

Radiological appearance

Ultrasound scans can be easily carried out and may give a vital early clue by showing midline shift (away from the side of the dilated pupil). A large tentorial haematoma can be visualized as an echodensity, as can a large convexity haematoma. Ventricular dilatation may occur secondary to aqueduct compression from a tentorial tear. However, US cannot give good visualization of the surface of the hemispheres, and CT is the preferred method when there is a high index of suspicion in a sick infant. Accurate localization of the haematoma is a great advantage if therapeutic tapping is to be carried out. Intensive care can be easily maintained throughout the relatively brief examination and no special sequences are required. Figure 5.21 shows images from the CT and MRI investigations of a term infant with seizures.

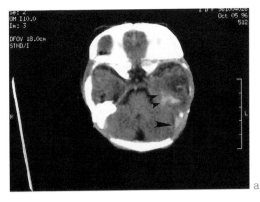

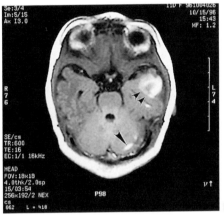

Fig. 5.21 Investigation of a term infant who presented with seizures. The CT scan (a) shows a linear hyperdense area (arrow) in the left subdural region adjacent to the left cerebellum consistent with a subdural haemorrhage. There is also patchy increased and decreased density in the left temporal lobe (double arrows) consistent with an intraparenchymal haemorrhage as well. Film (b) is an MRI taken 10 days later. It confirms the presence of both the subdural (arrow) and the intraparenchymal (double arrows) haemorrhages, which are seen as areas of increased signal intensity.

SPINAL CORD PATHOLOGY

Congenital abnormalities

Spina bifida is the term that covers defects of closure of the distal neural tube. It includes clinically obvious lesions such as myelomeningocele and meningocele, and more subtle variations such as spina bifida occulta.

- Myelomeningocele is a midline swelling of the spine which contains not only meninges but also spinal cord and cauda equina. This lesion is part of the Arnold–Chiari malformation type 2, and 80–90% develop hydrocephalus.
- Meningocele is a midline swelling which contains meninges and CSF but no spinal cord tissue.
- Spina bifida occulta refers to a vertebral anomaly with absence of a spinous process with varying involvement of the meninges and spinal cord. It may be associated with a lipoma, dermoid or diastematomyelia in which the spinal cord is split in two by fibrous tissue.

One clinical clue to an anomaly of the spinal cord may be abnormal hair growth or dimple over one region of the spine. Degrees of lower limb paresis may be present.

Clinical examination will show if and where the infant has loss of motor and sensory function. A plain X-ray will give some information but MRI gives the most complete information. This is particularly important in assessing infants with closed lesions such as diastematomyelia. Such infants may be neurologically intact initially but may lose function later as a result of tethering of the spinal cord. This is one situation where prophylactic neurosurgery is called for before irreversible loss of neurological function.

An example of a meningocele is shown in Chapter 9.

Trauma to the spinal cord

The spinal cord may be injured by excessive traction or rotation, usually in association with forceps or breech delivery. The typical clinical picture is of an infant who requires resuscitation at birth and reveals flaccid paralysis in the extremities. Sometimes the arms are less affected than the legs and there is paradoxical diaphragmatic movement without intercostal or abdominal muscle activity. If there is no significant brain lesion, the infant may show facial, mouth and eye movements. Occasionally the clinical picture resembles Werdnig–Hoffmann disease (infantile spinal muscular atrophy), but the clinical demonstration of a sensory level can indicate the spinal lesion. Ultrasonography will often demonstrate echogenicity in the damaged cord, and has the great advantage of being immediately available and avoiding movement of the sick infant. Later MRI can be used to give greater definition.

Figure 5.22 shows films from the investigation of a quadriplegic neonate born after a forceps delivery; forceps marks were seen on the forehead and neck.

VEIN OF GALEN MALFORMATION

Vein of Galen malformation is an aneurysmal dilatation of the vein into which drain anterior and middle cerebral arteries as well as other vessels. The clinical presentation is most commonly with cardiac failure in the neonatal period with an intracranial bruit and bounding carotid pulses. Seizures and hydrocephalus are not uncommon. Secondary brain damage may occur from 'steal' giving ischaemia or thrombosis. This lesion has a very high mortality rate without treatment but is important to recognize because successful therapy using embolization is now a possibility. Ultrasonography shows a large echolucent structure in the midline, and duplex Doppler can indicate the extent of the blood flow disturbance. A CT scan with contrast or MRI demonstrates this type of lesion well, but angiography will usually be required to plan therapy. Figure 5.23 is a series of images from two infants with vein of Galen malformations.

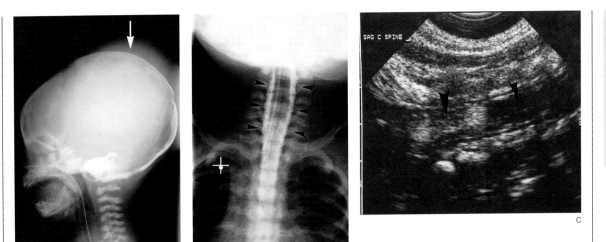

Fig. 5.22 Investigation of a quadriplegic neonate born after a forceps delivery. A plain film (a) of the skull shows only a large caput (arrow). The films of the cervical spine (not shown) were normal. A myelogram (b) shows only a minor cord enlargement, due to emergence of cord roots (arrows) in the cervical spine, which is normal. An US scan of the cervical spine (c) shows an echogenic area (larger arrow) in the upper cervical spine consistent with haemorrhage. This compares with the normal hypoechoic cord seen just inferior (smaller arrow).

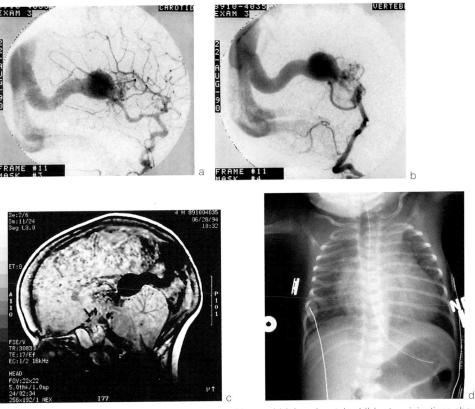

Fig. 5.23 Vein of Galen malformation. A cerebral angiogram with carotid (a) and vertebral (b) artery injections shows normal carotid and vertebral arteries with anastomoses to a grossly enlarged vein of Galen. The same infant is shown in (c) which is a sagittal image from an MRI examination showing the grossly enlarged vein of Galen. The CXR (d) from another infant with a vein of Galen malformation who presented with cardiac failure is typical of cardiac failure with cardiomegaly and increased pulmonary vascularity.

References

De Vries L S, Ekon S P, Dubowitz L M S 1992 The spectrum of leukomalacias using cranial ultrasound. Behavioural Brain Research 49: 1–6

Levene M I 1981 Measurement of the growth of the lateral ventricles in preterm infants with real time ultrasound. Archives of Disease in Childhood 56: 900–904

Lui K, Boag G, Danaman A, Costello S, Kirpalani H, Whyte H 1990 Widened subarachnoid space in pre-discharge cranial ultrasound: evidence of cerebral atrophy in immature infants? Development Medicine Child Neurology 32: 882–887

Ment L R, Duncan C C, Geehr R 1981 Benign enlargement of the subarachnoid spaces in the infant. Journal of Neurosurgery 54: 504–508

Pape K, Wigglesworth J 1979 Haemorrhage, ischemia and the perinatal brain. Clinics in Developmental Medicine No. 67/70. Spastics International Medical Publications, London

Pidcock F S, Graziani L J, Stanley C, Mitchell D G, Merton D 1990 Neurosonographic features of periventricular echodensities associated with cerebral palsy in preterm infants. Journal of Pediatrics 116: 417–422

Sarnat H B, Sarnat M S 1976 Neonatal encephalography following fetal distress. A clinical and electroencephalographic study. Archives of Neurology 33: 696–705

Ventriculomegaly Trial Group 1990 Randomised trial of early tapping in neonatal posthaemorrhagic ventricular dilatation. Archives of Disease in Childhood 65: 3–10

CHAPTER 6

The kidney

Haresh Kirpalani
John Mernagh
Gerald Gill

PRINCIPLES

The imaging of the neonatal kidney is usually prompted either by a routine antenatal assessment (see Chapter 9) or by well-defined clinical syndromes or signs. These signs are:

- oliguria – defined as < 1 ml/kg body weight of urine flow per hour after the first day of life
- renal failure – progressive azotaemia (urea > 20–30 mg/dl or 3.3–5.0 mmol/l) or elevated/rising creatinine levels (> 2.0 mg/dl or 180 μmol/l) after the first 3 days of life (Coulthard & Vernon 1995)
- haematuria
- renal masses found by manual palpation or by routine antenatal ultrasound
- hypertension
- evidence of overwhelming sepsis and/or a poor urine stream (giving concerns of obstructive uropathy)
- Potter's syndrome (pulmonary failure with oligohydramnios and contractures, etc. – see Chapter 9).

MODALITIES OF IMAGING

The clinical value of newborn renal imaging can be thought of as twofold: firstly, to provide detailed anatomical information, and secondly to provide functional information, as ancillary to clinical tests of renal function. Imaging of the newborn kidney has been difficult in the past owing to the poor concentrating ability of the newborn kidney and the relatively lower glomerular filtration rate. These are associated with the completion of nephrogenesis at 34 weeks of gestational age (Guignard 1992). New combinations of imaging techniques have overcome the problems of concentrating ability and late nephrogenesis. The previous mainstay of imaging – renal contrast imaging with intravenous pyelourograms – had confused the two separate aims of structural and functional assessment.

Ultrasonography

Ultrasonography of the neonatal kidney is used to assess gross structural abnormality. At its most extreme this includes agenesis or severe hypoplasia. Where the infant has obvious features of VACTERL (Vertebral, Anal, Cardiac, Tracheo-oEsophageal, Renal, Limb) anomalies, ultrasound imaging of the kidney will exclude any renal components of the complex. Although it is often advocated that spontaneous pneumothorax or a single umbilical artery should prompt a renal ultrasound scan, the pick-up is too low from these clinical signs to act as a screen for further investigation. The ultrasonographic appearance of a normal neonatal kidney is shown in Figure 6.1.

Ultrasound will also provide the only functional assessment possible in utero, since filling of the renal pelvis and voiding can be observed as well as size. Normal ranges for kidney size in utero by gestational age give a reference value (Romero et al 1989). The advent of non-invasive imaging in utero led initially to overdiagnosis of obstructive uropathies. This is because the renal calyceal system and ureters may appear to be dilated, and unless adequate time is given for micturition and release of urine, the normal size of the calyces and ureters may not be observed.

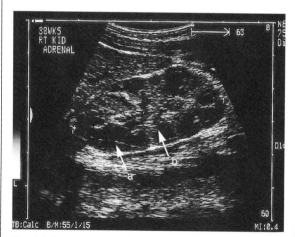

Fig. 6.1 Scan of a normal right neonatal kidney. The cortex is of similar echogenicity to the liver (arrow a). The renal pyramids are hypoechoic (arrow b).

Cystourethrograms

In settings of suspected uropathy with physical obstruction a voiding or retrograde cystourethrogram will be required. This will diagnose the likely sites: the ureteropelvic junction, insertion into the bladder at the trigone, the entrance of the urethra, and finally the posterior urethral valves and meatal stenosis (see Figs 6.13 and 6.8).

Renal scans

Renal function is assessed primarily by clinical means – urine flow and electrolyte and creatinine handling, and presence or absence of haematuria. However, renal flow studies using radioisotopes, most commonly diethylenetriamine pentaacetic acid (DTPA) labelled with ^{99m}Tc, provide ancillary information in difficult cases (Fig. 6.2).

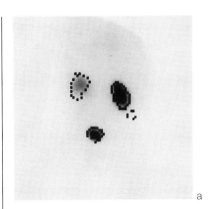

a

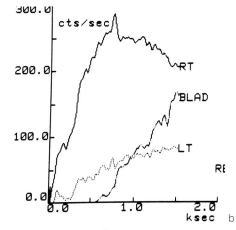

b

Fig. 6.2 A neonatal ^{99m}Tc-labelled DTPA scan in a baby aged 2 months known to have left hydronephrosis. Film (a) shows significantly less activity in the abnormal left kidney compared with the normal right kidney (scan taken posteriorly with the right kidney on the right side of the image). Film (b) shows the renal function curves: the right kidney shows normal function; the left kidney shows decreased function. The axes are counts/s for the y axis and time in ksec for the x axis.

RENAL FAILURE

Traditionally this is divided into pre-renal, renal and post-renal (generally obstructive) causes. Clinically, it should be possible to exclude distal obstructive uropathy (by examination of urinary stream and inspection for obvious deformities, and by gently passing a urinary catheter) and Potter's syndrome or absence of kidneys (see Fig. 2.75). The latter syndrome may present with mild degrees of renal failure, but is more likely to present with pulmonary failure. Many other renal conditions can present with renal failure; see the diagnostic categories below. However, two other important conditions need special consideration in the newborn: asphyxial renal damage from perinatal events, and renal venous thrombosis.

Perinatal asphyxia

Perinatal asphyxia is usually considered in the context of brain injury, but the syndrome entails multiorgan failure with myocardial necrosis (often papillary muscle necrosis), necrotizing enterocolitis and renal failure. A history of birth difficulties, with poor Apgar scores, is often obtained. A review of the fluid administration regimen will rule out simple prerenal dehydration. Renal damage in perinatal asphyxia is usually tubular and self-limited; anuria-oliguria and haematuria may be followed by spontaneous resolution. If the asphyxial insult is more profound, cortical necrosis may ensue, with more serious sequelae. These range from death through to recovery with cortical tissue loss and impaired renal function. Both medullary and cortical damage of this type may lead to heterotopic dysplastic calcification.

Radiological appearance The general ultrasonographic features of perinatal asphyxia in the kidneys are an overall increase in the echogenicity of the renal cortex and/or renal medulla with loss of corticomedullary differentiation. (Figs 6.3, 6.4). In mild to moderate asphyxia these findings usually resolve with time. The prognosis is generally worse when the cortex is severely affected rather than the medulla. This is the case in Figure 6.4 as opposed to the case in Figure 6.3.

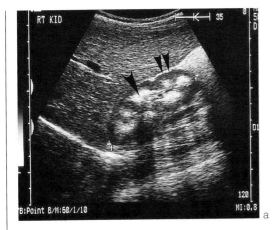

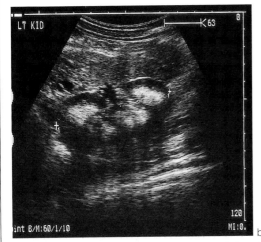

Fig. 6.3 Perinatal asphyxia: US images of the left and right kidneys (a, b) of a neonate with significantly increased echoes ('bright kidney') in the renal medulla (arrow) in comparison with the normal renal cortex (double arrows). Compare this with the normal neonatal kidney in Fig. 6.1.

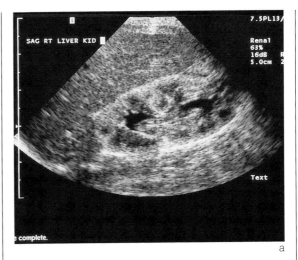

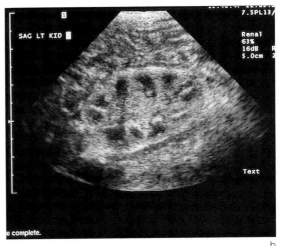

Fig. 6.4 US images of the right and left kidneys (a, b) of a neonate with significantly increased renal cortical echoes and loss of corticomedullary differentiation.

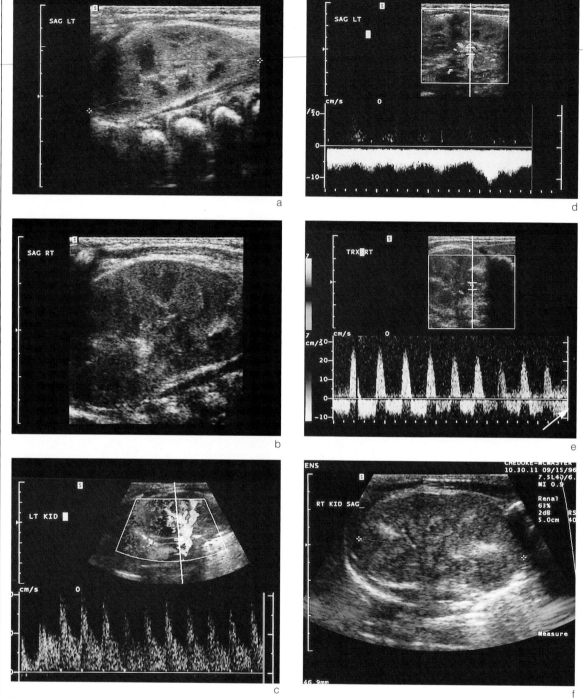

Fig. 6.5 (caption on p. 115)

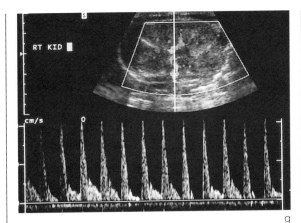

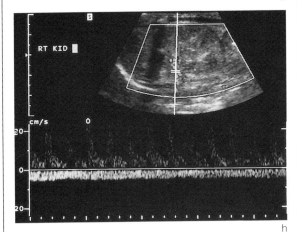

g

h

Fig. 6.5 Renal vein thrombosis. Ultrasound examination of a normal left kidney and an abnormal right kidney in a 1-day-old neonate. The left kidney (a) is normal, showing normal corticomedullary differentiation. The right kidney (b) is abnormal with a swollen, oedematous appearance and decreased corticomedullary differentiation. Doppler examination of the normal left renal artery (c) and the normal left renal vein (d) showed normal arterial and venous flow. Doppler examination of the right renal artery (e) showed arterial flow with reversed diastolic flow indicating increased resistance to arterial flow in the right kidney (i.e. below the zero line, see arrow). No venous flow was seen. Films f–h show the same patient 2 days later. The right kidney (f) appears less oedematous but still abnormal in appearance. Doppler examination of the right renal artery (g) now shows no reversed diastolic flow, indicating a more normal resistance to arterial flow. Doppler examination of the right renal vein (h) now shows normal or near-normal venous flow.

Renal vein thrombosis

Clinical features Renal vein thrombosis may follow dehydration (e.g. from vomiting or diarrhoea), asphyxia, sepsis or umbilical vein catheterization. There may be evidence of thromboembolic disease elsewhere in the body, such as inferior vena cava (IVC) thrombosis with oedema and swelling of the lower half of the body.

The best-recognized clinical entity is a triad of enlarged renal masses with haematuria and renal failure, but variations are common and are probably often unrecognized. Predisposing conditions include perinatal asphyxia and the presence of indwelling lines such as umbilical arterial and venous catheters (Schmidt 1995). The natural history is not well understood, but at its worst this condition may lead to severe renal failure with death, and at best to full 'spontaneous' resolution. This leads to difficulty in prescribing therapy. Treatment is usually conservative without anticoagulation, and in most cases renal function returns to normal.

Radiological appearance The ultrasound findings are of a smooth, enlarged kidney with loss of the normal corticomedullary differentiation, (Fig. 6.5). Doppler examination can show the decrease in venous return from the kidney. A thrombus can sometimes be noted in the IVC (Fig. 6.6).

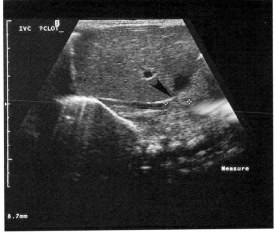

Fig. 6.6 Sagittal image of the IVC showing a probable small thrombus in the IVC. (See arrow for IVC and crosses for area of thrombus.)

AORTIC AND RENAL ARTERIAL THROMBOSIS

The presentation of aortic thrombosis is that of left heart outlet obstruction, as also seen in hypoplastic left heart syndromes. Renal arterial thrombus presents with hypertensive cardiac failure and haematuria. In both aortic and renal artery thrombosis the likely source of thrombus is an indwelling umbilical artery line. Both conditions may resolve spontaneously (Fig. 6.7). However, repeat US showing non-resolution with possible extension and/or hypertension may prompt more aggressive therapy. In severe renal arterial disease with catastrophic hypertension, therapy may require unilateral nephrectomy, if only to save the other kidney. The role of renal arterial contrast injections is controversial and many centres would avoid such investigations. The advent of Doppler scanning techniques avoids invasive examinations.

PRUNE-BELLY SYNDROME

Prune-belly syndrome is a congenital multisystem disorder seen almost exclusively in males. The clinical presentation is with a markedly absent abdominal musculature with evident massive abdominal distension, and there are associated urinary tract anomalies of megalocystis and megaloureter. A differential includes various causes of tense ascites. There may be other associated abnormalities including gastrointestinal abnormalities such as malrotation, intestinal atresia and imperforate anus.

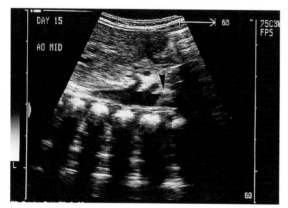

Fig. 6.7 Aortic thrombus showing complete block of the descending aorta (arrow). This resolved clinically and radiologically within 10 days with no anticoagulation.

Radiological appearance

The radiological features of prune-belly syndrome are those of the individual abnormalities, i.e. distended abdomen seen on plain films secondary to the absent abdominal wall muscles, dilated bladder and ureters seen on retrograde cystoureterogram secondary to megalocystis-megaloureter, and gastrointestinal abnormalities identified on upper and lower gastrointestinal tract examinations (Fig. 6.8).

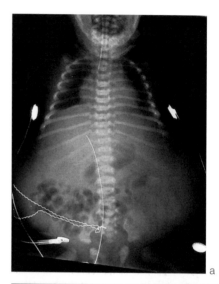

a

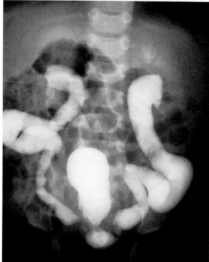

b

Fig. 6.8 Prune-belly syndrome. Plain film of the abdomen of a neonate with this syndrome shows the grossly distended abdomen secondary to the absent abdominal wall muscles. A retrograde cystoureterogram (b) shows grossly dilated ureters.

CYSTIC DISEASE

The nomenclature of the various cysts affecting the neonatal urogenital system is somewhat confusing. All of these conditions present with a combination of clinical features – the presence of masses, pulmonary failure and contractures. Masses may give dystocia with a difficult or obstructed labour. The degree of pulmonary failure and contractures depend upon the degree of intrauterine compromise of urine production. The presence or otherwise of a family history of renal masses or symptoms should be sought, although this is usually recognized after an infant is born with a cyst. The differentiation of the type of cystic disease will be assisted by the investigations outlined below.

Polycystic kidney disease

Clinical features There are two forms of polycystic kidney disease, the autosomal dominant (or adult polycystic kidney disease), and the autosomal recessive (or infantile polycystic kidney disease). Both usually present with renal masses in the newborn, or with renal failure. The autosomal recessive form involves an abnormal proliferation and dilatation of the collecting tubules resulting in multiple 1–2 mm cysts. Often there is a periportal fibrosis in the liver and pancreatic fibrosis. If lesions are seen in the liver this is diagnostic of this form. Commonly this condition is detected in the antenatal period, and early postnatal renal failure ensues. Oligohydramnios and large, echogenic kidneys may be seen on antenatal examination. In this presentation, the prognosis is poor with death from renal failure or respiratory insufficiency due to pulmonary hypoplasia.

Autosomal recessive polycystic kidney disease is far commoner than the autosomal dominant variant (so called adult variant). Both can present with renal failure within the first month of life. Again, the prognosis is poor, with renal failure, hypertension or left ventricular failure causing death within the first year of life.

Radiological appearance The ultrasound features of autosomal recessive polycystic kidney disease are of enlarged, echogenic kidneys which can be seen on both antenatal and postnatal scans (Fig. 6.9).

The adult form may be diagnosed from the parental history, or ultrasound scanning of the parent. Ultrasound distinction from the neonatal recessive form in the newborn alone, is not possible unless there is evidence of liver involvement, which does not occur with the adult form.

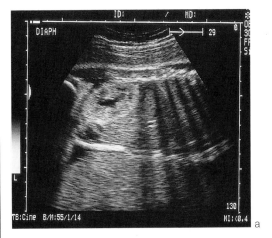

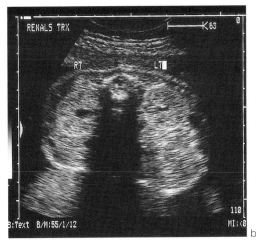

Fig. 6.9 Prenatal ultrasound examination showing the right (a) fetal kidney in the sagittal plane and both (b) fetal kidneys in the transverse plane. Both kidneys are large and echogenic, highly suggestive of autosomal recessive polycystic kidney disease.

Multicystic dysplastic kidney disease

Clinical features Multicystic dysplastic kidney disease is the second most common cause of abdominal mass in the neonate after hydronephrosis. An early extrarenal obstruction or atresia leads to an aberrant development of the collecting ducts and tubules and multiple cysts. There are often associated renal anomalies including ureteropelvic junction obstruction, horseshoe kidneys and ureteral anomalies including posterior urethral valves. Bilateral disease occurs in up to 20% of cases.

Radiological appearance The most common findings on ultrasonography are multiple, randomly placed cysts of various sizes with the largest cyst in a peripheral non-medial location (this differentiates multicystic kidneys from hydronephrosis with a dilated pelvis) (Fig. 6.10). When seen antenatally oligohydramnios is noted in bilateral disease or in unilateral disease with contralateral obstruction or agenesis.

OBSTRUCTIVE UROPATHY

Ureteropelvic junction obstruction

Some causes have already been discussed, such as the megalocystis and megaloureter syndromes. However, simple hydronephrosis is more common, and the most common cause is a ureteropelvic junction obstruction. These are often associated with infections. The radiological features are those of hydronephrosis without hydroureter, i.e. a large, dilated renal pelvis which communicates with enlarged dilated calyces. These features are important as they allow ureteropelvic obstruction to be distinguished from multicystic dysplastic kidney with which it is associated (Fig. 6.11).

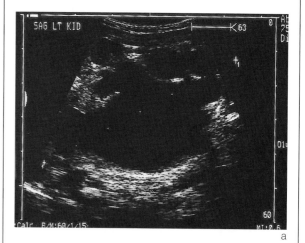

a

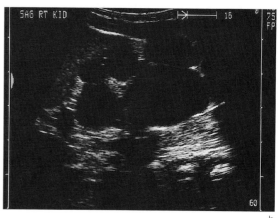

b

Fig. 6.11 A neonatal US examination shows hydronephrosis of the left kidney (a) with no associated hydroureter; this is compared with the right multiplastic dysplastic kidney, (b). Note communication of the pelvis and calyces in the left kidney but not in the right.

Fig. 6.10 Multicystic dysplastic kidney disease. Neonatal ultrasound scan shows that the left kidney has multiple cysts and no identifiable normal renal cortex or renal pelvis. The right kidney (not shown) was normal. A second example is shown in Fig. 6.11b.

Duplex collecting system

Duplication is the most common anomaly of the upper renal collecting system. A duplex collecting system can be unilateral or bilateral; it can be complete, with two separate renal pelves and ureters for each kidney, or partial. It may be associated with a ureterocele. Neonates with partial duplex collecting systems are usually asymptomatic. Patients with complete duplication, however, may present with signs of sepsis, usually of the upper pole system. The lower pole system usually does not become obstructed but may have associated vesicoureteral reflux. Associated abnormalities of obstruction can include prune-belly syndrome, renal dysplasia, pulmonary hypoplasia, and neonatal ascites, urothorax or urinoma as a result of urine leak.

Radiological appearance The usual radiological findings of a duplex collecting system are of obstruction of the upper pole ureter with hydronephrosis of the upper pole collecting system and associated hydroureter. A ureterocele is sometimes seen. The lower pole collecting system is usually seen to be normal (Fig. 6.12).

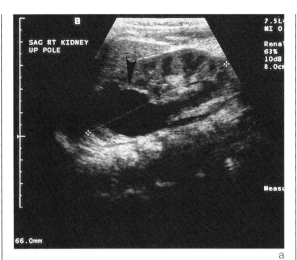

a

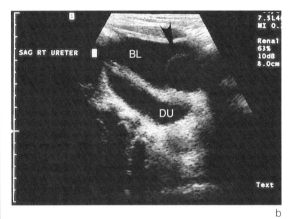

b

Fig. 6.12 Ultrasound examination of a neonate with a duplex collecting system on the right. There is obstruction of the upper pole system (a) with a dilated upper pole renal pelvis (arrow). The lower pole collecting system is normal. The upper pole ureter is dilated down to the bladder (b). An associated ureterocele was present projecting into the bladder (b, arrow). BL, bladder; DU, dilated ureter.

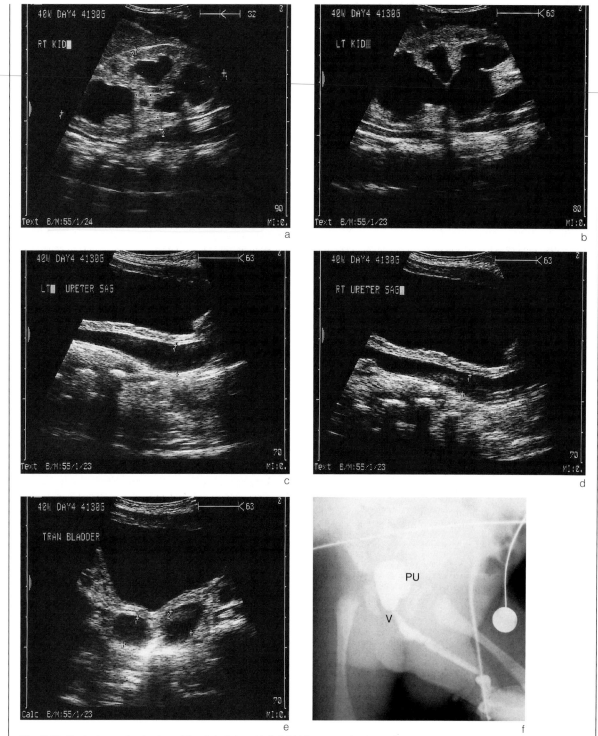

Fig. 6.13 Posterior urethral valves. The right (a) and left (b) kidneys are hydronephrotic with grossly distended renal pelves and calyces. Bilateral hydroureters are shown, with the right and left ureters seen in the sagittal (c, d) and transverse (e) planes. In the sagittal plane these are seen as long, tubular structures extending from the renal pelves down to the bladder trigone. The bladder is also dilated, in keeping with an obstruction at the level of the urethra. A retrograde urethrogram (f) shows a normal-diameter anterior urethra but a grossly dilated posterior urethra (PU) indicative of posterior urethral valves (V).

Posterior urethral valves

Posterior urethral valves are congenital thick folds of mucous membrane located in the posterior urethra. This is the most common cause of urethral obstruction in the male infant and presentation may be with a poor urine stream, or in an emergency with sepsis and shock. Prenatally, bladder outlet obstruction may be seen with oligohydramnios and an overdistended bladder or bilateral hydronephrosis and hydroureter. Hypoplastic or dysplastic kidneys may also be associated with posterior urethral valves.

Radiological appearance The radiological features of posterior urethral valves are those of obstruction at the level of the urethra: hydronephrosis and hydroureter with a distended bladder. The valves can sometimes be visualized on retrograde urethrography as a thin valve across the urethra. Figure 6.13f shows simply a 'ballooning', and Figure 6.13a–e are films from an ultrasound examination in a neonate with posterior urethral valves.

RENAL CANDIDIASIS

Candida has become increasingly recognized as a cause of nosocomial infection. Two cases are shown here: one case shows obvious renal involvement (Fig. 6.14), and the other shows no renal involvement although the child died in overwhelming fungaemia (Fig. 6.15). At autopsy hyphae were present throughout the body including the kidneys of this latter patient. The vector of *Candida* is often maternal in early presentations, and the disease may present as a congenital pneumonia. In later cases the vector may be the caregivers or colonizing skin flora. Multiple courses of antibiotics may diminish host resistance. Presentation is usually that of a non-specific 'sepsis'. Prophylactic nystatin to the mouth is indicated in the very low-birthweight infant. The diagnosis may be suspected, but a positive blood culture may be the first indication. The key to diagnosis is a high level of suspicion and any positive cultures should not be lightly dismissed as

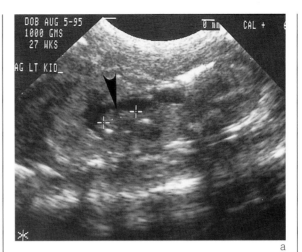

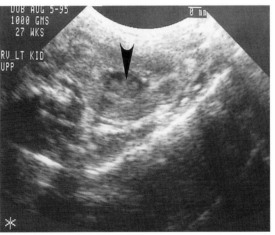

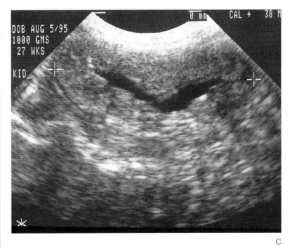

Fig. 6.14 Renal candidiasis. Sagittal (a) and transverse (b) images from a neonatal US examination showing a rounded echogenic lesion, the fungus ball, in the left renal pelvis (arrows). After treatment with amphotericin this resolved (c).

'contaminants'. If a positive blood culture is found, an active search at other sites is needed, including two-dimensional echocardiography, eye examination by an ophthalmologist searching for retinal fungal foci, renal ultrasonography and cerebrospinal fluid analysis for meningeal involvement.

Radiological appearance

The fungal balls of renal candidiasis can be seen on ultrasonography as echogenic, non-shadowing masses in the renal pelvis and calices. They cannot be readily distinguished from other non-shadowing masses in the renal pelvis such as blood clots. Negative radiological findings must be weighed with clinical findings.

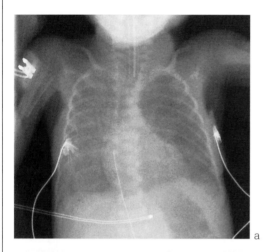

a

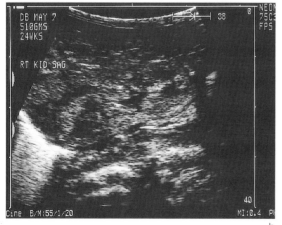

b

Fig. 6.15 Renal candidiasis. The CXR (a) shows only a mild diffuse shadowing which was attributed to 'chronic lung disease'. The kidneys appeared normal on US (b).

The baby of birth weight 500 g shown in Figure 6.15 had several predispositions for generalized candidiasis: multiple long lines with difficulty in access, multiple courses of antibiotics, and chronic ventilation. The CXR shows mild diffuse shadowing suggesting respiratory distress syndrome. However, at postmortem the lung was found to be loaded with fungal hyphae despite 'blind' anticandidal therapy with amphotericin and 5-fluorocytosine. The same was true of the kidneys. On ultrasonography the kidneys had appeared normal.

NEPHROCALCINOSIS

The diagnosis of nephrocalcinosis is usually suspected from the history rather than from clinical signs, or it may be noted as part of an ultrasound examination. Commonly it results from prolonged courses of frusemide (UK) (furosemide in USA) in bronchopulmonary dysplasia. Over time, calciuria leads to deposition in the kidneys. An alternative cause is healing of severe asphyxia by metastatic calcification, or the condition may be part of a congenital problem such as renal tubular acidosis or renal cystic disease. Therapy is not usually required in the newborn period, although when appropriate, frusemide should be stopped. Later on there may be renal insufficiency, although some cases regress.

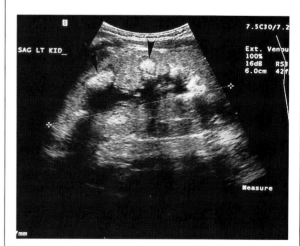

Fig. 6.16 Neonatal nephrocalcinosis. Note the increased echogenicity in the renal pyramids (arrows) compared with the renal cortex. There is posterior shadowing from the echogenic pyramids in keeping with nephrocalcinosis.

Radiological appearance

On ultrasonography neonatal nephrocalcinosis is seen as increased echogenicity in the renal pyramids with normal-appearing renal cortex (Fig. 6.16).

ADRENAL HAEMORRHAGE

In the newborn adrenal haemorrhage is associated with birth trauma or, less commonly, haemorrhagic disorders. It is therefore seen within the first week of life. It is bilateral in 10% of cases. Adrenal haemorrhage is detected with ultrasound: an echogenic mass is seen which becomes hypoechoic as the haemorrhage resolves. It may later calcify.

Figure 6.17 shows an example of an adrenal haemorrhage superior to the right kidney. On this examination the haemorrhage is seen as a rounded lesion of mixed but primarily low echogenicity measuring approximately 2 cm in diameter. A comparison is made with the left adrenal gland, which looks normal with a thin, elongated, well-defined appearance. Incidental note was made of the fact that the left kidney was absent in this neonate, making the left adrenal gland easier to visualize.

URACHAL ABNORMALITIES

Embryologically there is a normal communication between the apex of the bladder and the umbilicus, which closes prior to birth. Persistence of this communication can result in a persistent urachus with resulting passage of urine from the bladder to the umbilicus. A urachal diverticulum results in the presence of the urachus at the bladder end. A urachal cyst (Fig. 6.18) results from the persistence of a fluid-filled urachus closed at both the bladder and umbilical ends. These may become infected.

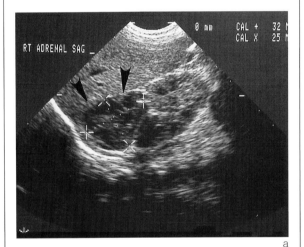

Fig. 6.17 Adrenal haemorrhage. (a) Right adrenal haemorrhage appears as an area of mixed but primarily low echogenicity measuring approximately 2 cm in diameter (arrows). The left adrenal gland (b) appears normal (arrows).

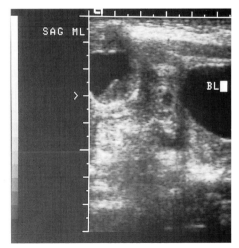

Fig. 6.18 Urachal cyst. Sagittal ultrasound image of the pelvis of a neonate. The bladder is identified on the right (BL). Just superior to the bladder there is a cystic structure with some debris seen within it: this is a urachal cyst.

References

Coulthard M, Vernon B 1995 Managing acute renal failure in very low birthweight infants. Arch Dis Child Fetal Neonatal Ed 73: F187–F192

Guignard J P 1992 in Fetal and neonatal physiology, vol. 2, Ch. 118. Philadelphia, Saunders).

Romero R, Pilu G, Jeanty P et al 1989 Prenatal diagnosis of congenital anomalies. East Norwalk, Appleton & Lang

Schmidt B, Andrew M 1995 Neonatal thrombosis: report of a retrospective Canadian and International registry. Pediatrics 96: 939–943

CHAPTER 7

Bone

Aideen Moore
Gerald Gill
Haresh Kirpalani

PRINCIPLES

Imaging studies of bone in the newborn infant are most often undertaken for evaluation of congenital abnormalities, for suspected trauma, and in the investigation of infections, either congenital or acquired.

MODALITIES OF IMAGING

Plain film radiography remains the principal method of evaluating the newborn suspected of bony abnormality. In most instances both anteroposterior (AP) and lateral views are required. Proper positioning and immobilization of the neonate are important for good studies. 'Babygrams' (a film of the whole infant) are useful in documenting proportions and to give an overall view of the skeleton, then allowing one to choose more localized views.

Ultrasound studies are becoming increasingly valuable, particularly in screening for hip dysplasia. Ultrasound is also useful when spinal cord injuries are suspected. With more frequent antenatal ultrasound scans, abnormalities of bone can sometimes be suspected and diagnosed in utero.

Bone scanning in the neonate is primarily used when osteomyelitis is suspected; however, owing to the high vascularity and metabolism of bones in the newborn infant, it is not as useful as at other times of life.

Neither computed tomography (CT) nor magnetic resonance imaging (MRI) has a major role to play in evaluation of the skeletal system in the neonate, except in planning complex corrective cranial surgery (see Fig. 7.22).

SKELETAL DYSPLASIAS

The skeletal dysplasias comprise a large group of mainly single-gene disorders of cartilage and/or bone growth that frequently produce disproportionate short stature. Many of these dysplasias are recognized at birth, some even antenatally, because of abnormal bone echodensity on fetal ultrasound examination. Over a hundred distinct disorders have been described, and many can be diagnosed using clinical and radiographic criteria alone. Differential diagnosis entails taking a detailed family history, making an assessment of body proportions (e.g. short-limb dwarfism or short-trunk dwarfism) and an assessment of the limb segment involved. Many skeletal dysplasias are associated with fractures, while others have associated anomalies. Important reference books such as *Smith's Recognizable patterns of human malformation* (Jones 1997) and *Caffey's Pediatric X-ray diagnosis* (Silverman & Kuhn 1993) should be available in the neonatal unit. Final diagnosis is often through the combined efforts of neonatologist, clinical geneticist, gene analyst and radiologist. In spite of this it is not always possible to make a specific diagnosis. Only a few of the major abnormalities can be discussed here.

Thanatophoric dysplasia

Thanatophoric dysplasia is the most common lethal bone dysplasia; nevertheless it is still rare, with an incidence of 1 in 40 000 births. There is severe shortening of the extremities and a narrow chest. Infants are stillborn or die shortly after birth owing to pulmonary hypoplasia. The characteristic radiographic appearance is shown in Figures 7.1 and 7.2.

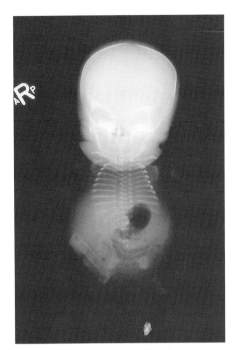

Fig. 7.1 Thanatophoric dysplasia. The X-ray shows a normal-sized head, out of proportion to the small body and short limbs. Unlike osteogenesis imperfecta or hypophosphatasia the skull is well mineralized. The extremely short ribs and pulmonary hypoplasia make this a lethal condition.

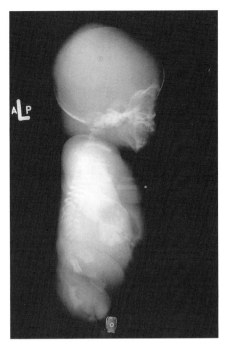

Fig. 7.2 Thanatophoric dysplasia. The inverted U-shaped lumbar vertebrae and 'telephone receiver' femurs, seen here best on the lateral film, characterize this condition.

Osteogenesis imperfecta

There are several forms of osteogenesis imperfecta, characterized by increased bone fragility because of connective tissue abnormalities, primarily defects in type I collagen. Owing to the defective bone cortex and spongiosa, the bones are weak and fracture easily. The autosomal recessive or perinatal form is lethal. Since it is often sporadic or a new mutant, there may be no prior family history. Infants are stillborn or die shortly after birth owing to pulmonary hypoplasia. Clinically they have numerous fractures. The differential diagnosis includes many of the skeletal dysplasias; if the infant has been at home, non-accidental injury (NAI) may be considered, but quickly ruled out.

Examples of this condition are shown in Figures 7.3–7.6.

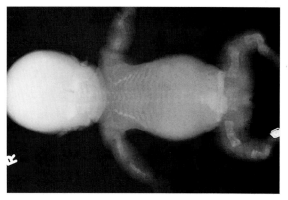

Fig. 7.5 Postnatal X-ray of stillborn baby. In osteogenesis imperfecta all the bones are poorly mineralized, including the skull. The thorax is narrow and hypoplastic (bell-shaped). The spine is often relatively normal. The long bones and ribs are distorted with multiple fractures which have occurred throughout intrauterine life and are thus at different stages of evolution.

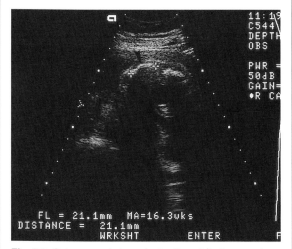

Fig. 7.3 Osteogenesis imperfecta. Prenatal ultrasound scan at 24 weeks gestation shows a thickened, short femur. Estimated gestational age based on the femur length was 16.3 weeks.

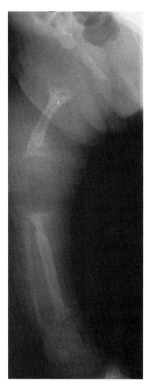

Fig. 7.6 This localized view of the femur and tibia shows multiple fractures, some of which are healing.

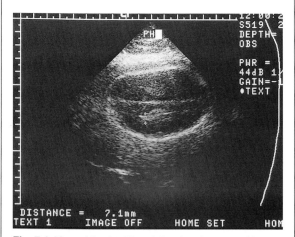

Fig. 7.4 View of the fetal head showing the ease with which the head can be deformed with pressure from the transducer as a result of poor ossification of the cranium.

Achondroplasia

Achondroplasia in the newborn period is primarily a short-limbed dwarfism. It is the most common non-lethal bone dysplasia. It is mainly a disorder of cartilage, thus bones initially formed in cartilage (endochondral) are most affected. The transmission is autosomal dominant but the heterozygous form may be sporadic in up to 80% of cases. Homozygous individuals show the most severe features of achondroplasia with disproportionate limb shortening, more marked proximally (rhizomelic) than distally. Infants with the homozygous form are often stillborn or succumb in the neonatal period, usually from respiratory failure.

The radiographic appearance is illustrated in Figures 7.7–7.9.

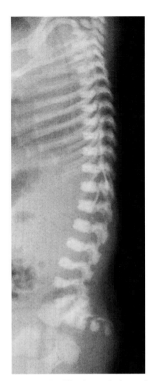

Fig. 7.8 Achondroplasia. The lateral view of the spine shows the characteristic lumbosacral lordosis.

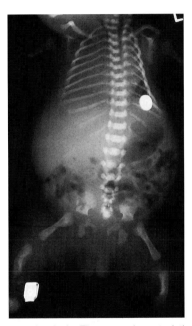

Fig. 7.7 Achondroplasia. There are characteristic spinal abnormalities, the spinal pedicles come closer together in the lumbosacral region and the pelvis is reduced in size because of undergrowth of the ilia.

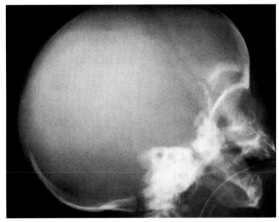

Fig. 7.9 Achondroplasia. The skull is well mineralized. The face is small in proportion to the skull.

Metaphyseal dysplasia

Metaphyseal dysplasia is another form of short-limbed dwarfism. The spine and bone length are relatively normal, but the metaphyses are flared and irregular (Figs 7.10, 7.11).

Multiple epiphyseal dysplasia

Multiple epiphyseal dysplasia is a type of short-limbed dwarfism with a very characteristic radiographic appearance. This disease presents with mild limb shortening, leading to premature joint disease in later life. The epiphyses ossify from multiple centres resulting in stippled calcification, causing a distorted epiphysis as growth occurs (Figs 7.12, 7.13).

Osteopetrosis

Osteopetrosis is a disease of defective osteoclast function with failure of proper resorption and remodelling resulting in sclerotic, thick, brittle bone. Because of the defective osteoclast activity the original bone is not remodelled, leading to the 'bone within a bone' appearance (Figs 7.14, 7.15). All cell lineages in the bone marrow are affected, with consequent development of haematopoiesis in extramedullary sites. The infantile autosomal recessive form presents with failure to thrive, hepatosplenomegaly, lymphadenopathy, anaemia, leukopenia and thrombocytopenia.

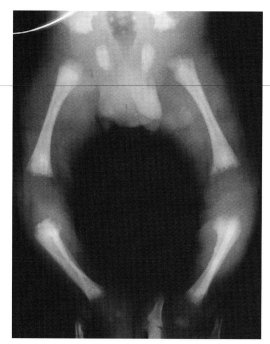

Fig. 7.10 The lower limbs of an infant with the characteristic changes of metaphyseal dysplasia in both the proximal and distal metaphyses.

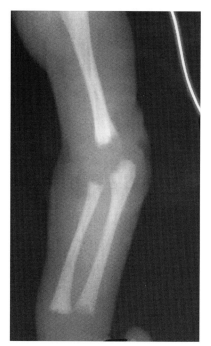

Fig. 7.11 Metaphyseal dysplasia. Upper limbs of the infant in Fig. 7.10.

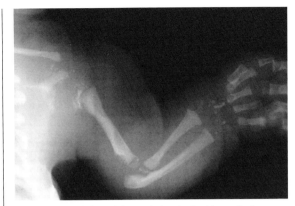

Fig. 7.12 Multiple epiphyseal dysplasia. Upper limb, showing shortened bones and stippled epiphyses.

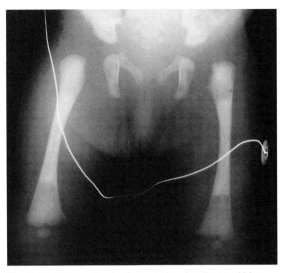

Fig. 7.14 Osteopetrosis. Femurs showing 'bone within a bone'.

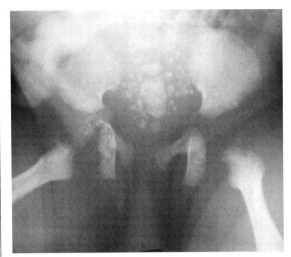

Fig. 7.13 Multiple epiphyseal dysplasia. Pelvis, showing multiple ossification sites throughout the sacrum, and right pelvic ramus.

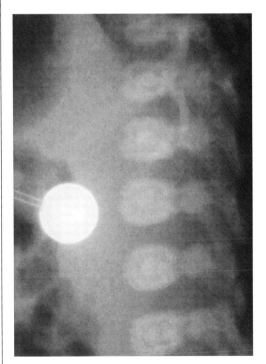

Fig. 7.15 Osteopetrosis. The same appearance is shown in the lateral view of the spine.

Hypophosphatasia

Hypophosphatasia is characterized by poor mineralization of bone with low activity of serum, bone and liver alkaline phosphatases (Figs 7.16, 7.17). It is a rare autosomal recessive disorder. In the neonatal or congenital lethal form, there is marked demineralization of the calvarium and lack of calcification of the metaphyseal ends of long bones. Cupping of metaphyses is also noted. The prognosis is poor, with death usually seen within 6 months.

ACQUIRED LESIONS OF BONE

Osteopenia of prematurity

Osteopenia of prematurity (Fig. 7.18), previously known as rickets of prematurity, occurs primarily in very low-birthweight infants. The disorder is largely prevented by dietary supplementation with calcium and phosphorus, or the use of specialized premature formulae, and is rarely seen in the nursery today, although it does still occur in infants receiving prolonged courses of total parenteral nutrition. Previously, and especially in the case of premature infants with chronic lung disease, it was often manifested by numerous rib fractures. Nowadays, if it occurs it is most commonly seen as bone undermineralization. It is possible to quantify this in the research setting by bone densitometry. Biochemically it is often noted that the level of alkaline phosphatase is elevated, serum calcium is usually normal, while serum phosphate is decreased. Rickets is defined as osteomalacia occurring during the period of endochondral bone growth (Fig. 7.19). True fetal or congenital rickets is rare; it may result from severe maternal nutritional osteomalacia associated with calcium and vitamin D deficiency.

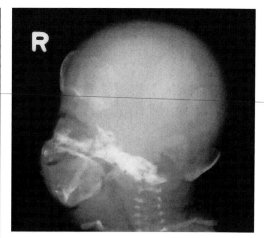

Fig. 7.16 Hypophosphatasia. The skull is characteristic with small, extremely poorly mineralized bones.

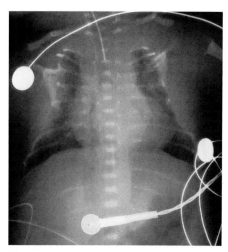

Fig. 7.17 Hypophosphatasia. The spine and ribs are also very poorly mineralized. Rib fractures are seen, with consequent distortion.

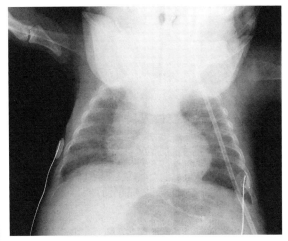

Fig. 7.18 Osteopenia of prematurity. CXR showing generalized bone undermineralization with semi-translucent ribs, vertebral bodies and long bones. This is a long-term neonate with a ventricular–peritoneal shunt in place and some chronic lung disease.

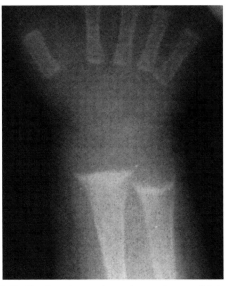

Fig. 7.19 The flared, cup-shaped metaphyses of rickets.

Thyroid disorders

In uncontrolled maternal hyperthyroidism the infant may present with hyperthyroidism. In addition to the generalized features of hyperthyroidism (see Chapter 3), the bone findings are secondary to those of advanced calcification in ossification centres that should not be ossified (Fig. 7.20).

Infantile hypothyroidism may be diagnosed on congenital screening, or more rarely suspected clinically. Congenital hypothyroidism will result in delayed bone ossification, which in the term newborn is evidenced by failure of tibial epiphyseal ossification.

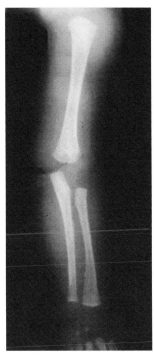

Fig. 7.20 Even at 32 weeks gestational age, epiphyses that are usually not present at birth can be seen: these are the proximal humeral as well as the capitate and hamate at the wrist. Normally the humeral centre is present at birth to 3 months, and the wrist epiphyses at 3–6 months.

Craniosynostosis

Craniosynostosis is a premature closure of the cranial sutures. It encompasses a wide spectrum of disorders, depending on which suture or sutures are fused. The spectrum ranges from mild cosmetic abnormalities through to severe microcephaly.

Clinical features Deformities are palpable and often visible. Sagittal craniosynostosis produces a long scaphocephalic (boat-shaped) head with bulging frontal bones and a palpable ridge along the line of the fused suture. Coronal synostosis leads to a short, high head with a flattened forehead, often unilateral. This may be associated with a recognizable craniofacial dysmorphic syndrome such as Apert's or Crouzon's disease. Identify cases of craniosynostosis as soon as possible because results of early corrective surgery are superior. Where only a single suture is involved this may not be so crucial, except from the cosmetic point of view.

Radiological appearance A plain skull X-ray may confirm the diagnosis, but with sagittal and coronal suture involvement or in craniofacial syndromes there is a risk of raised intracranial pressure and hydrocephalus. Detailed imaging with CT or MRI is indicated (Figs 7.21, 7.22).

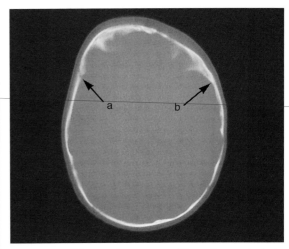

Fig. 7.21 A CT scan of a neonate with craniosynostosis. In this example the left coronal suture is fused (arrow a) and there is flattening of the left frontal and parietal area. The right coronal suture has a normal appearance (arrow b).

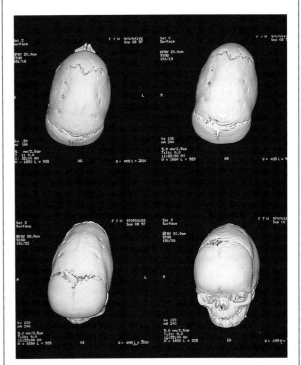

Fig. 7.22 Using computer programming the bone windows from the CT images are put together to form a three-dimensional view, which can be viewed from various angles. These reconstructed images show that the sagittal suture is absent. The skull appears long and narrow. The coronal, metopic and lambdoid sutures are present.

Limb anomalies

The extremities, especially the hands, can display a wide variety of malformations, such as syndactyly, polydactyly and brachydactyly, which may occur in isolation or as part of different syndromes. The most common is syndactyly, fusion or webbing of two digits. Simple syndactyly involves skin and soft tissue, whereas complex syndactyly involves various degrees of osseous fusion (Fig. 7.23).

Hypoplasia of the thumbs can be seen in Holt–Oram syndrome, an autosomal dominant defect which is often associated with cardiac abnormalities, usually an atrial septal defect; or, as in Figure 7.24, in de Lange's syndrome.

Hemivertebrae

Hemivertebrae can occur either singly or as part of a larger syndrome such as the VACTERL anomalies (see p. 64). They occur as a result of malformation of the two ossification centres for the ventral and dorsal halves of the vertebral bones (Fig. 7.25). There may also be associated scoliosis.

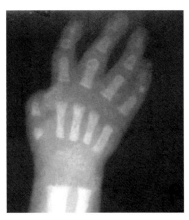

Fig. 7.24 Upper limb X-rays of an infant with de Lange's syndrome.

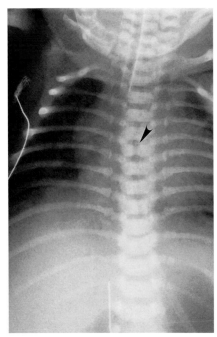

Fig. 7.25 Thoracic hemivertebrae. This malformation can be very subtle, as seen here (arrow).

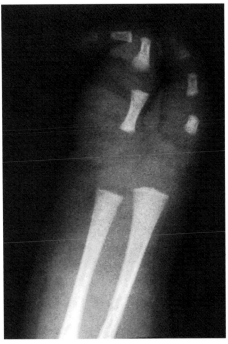

Fig. 7.23 'Lobster claw' hands with the digits located medially and laterally.

Caudal regression syndrome

There are varying degrees of hypoplasia to aplasia of the lower spine and sacrum. The example shown in Figure 7.26 is of complete absence of the lumbar spine and sacrum.

Congenital hip dislocation

Congenital dislocation of the hip (CDH), or congenital dysplasia of the hip, develops because of abnormal ligament laxity. This is believed to be an effect of maternal oestrogen. Infants born in the breech position with hyperflexion of the hips resulting in shortening of the iliopsoas muscle are more likely to develop hip dysplasia. Other infants at risk include those with evidence of positional deformation such as skull moulding deformities, infants with neuromuscular disorders, congenital torticollis, or a family history of congenital hip dysplasia. Diagnosis is suspected on clinical examination when the hip is found to be dislocated or dislocatable, using the Ortolani and Barlow manoeuvres. Ultrasound scans of the affected hip, both at rest and during movement, are valuable methods of identifying and monitoring CDH (Fig. 7.27). Many cases of dislocatable hips resolve spontaneously, thus there is much debate surrounding diagnosis and management (Foster 1995).

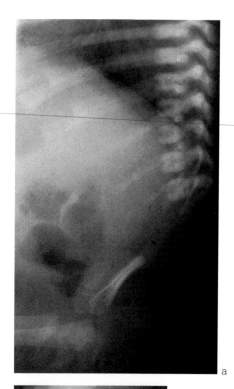

a

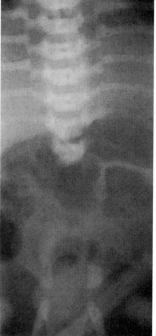

b

Fig. 7.26 Frontal (a) and lateral (b) views of the lower spine of a neonate with caudal regression syndrome. The lumbar spine and sacrum are absent. The iliac bones have moved medially.

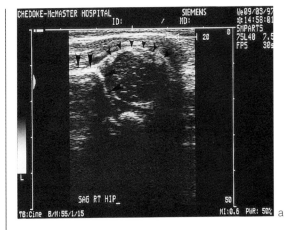

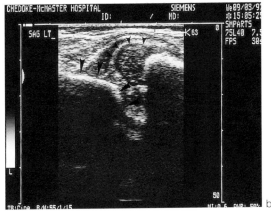

Fig. 7.27 Ultrasonograms of congenital dysplasia of the hip. (a) Sagittal US image from the normal right hip; note the normal-appearing iliac spine and roof of the acetabulum (large arrows). The femoral head is well aligned in the acetabulum (small arrows). (b) Sagittal US image from the abnormal left hip. The acetabulum is shallower than on the right with some flattening of the acetabular roof (large arrows). The femoral head is subluxed superiorly and laterally (small arrows).

Osteomyelitis

Acute osteomyelitis most commonly affects children. In the newborns the usual organisms are *staphylococcus aureus*, group B streptococcus, coagulase-negative staphylococcus and *Escherichia coli*. The source of the infection is most commonly blood-borne, genitourinary or dermal, which may be related to the siting of indwelling lines. Most commonly the lower extremity is involved. In the neonatal period there is often little or no systemic disturbance. Swelling or paucity of movement of the affected limb may be observed. Multicentric involvement is common, often with both joint involvement and septic arthritis. In the infant, infection can spread across the epiphysis because transfascial vessels cross the growth plate into the epiphysis. White cell counts are usually raised with a left shift and elevated levels of C-reactive protein. Blood cultures should also be obtained. Radiographs are usually negative at first, only later showing the characteristic periosteal changes. The bone scan can also be falsely negative or equivocal in up to 70%.

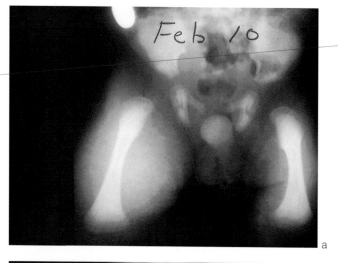

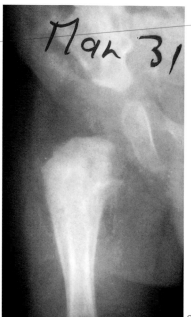

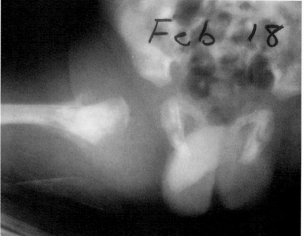

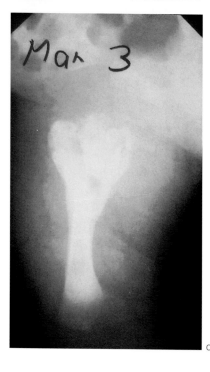

Fig. 7.28 Osteomyelitis and septic arthritis. (a) Soft tissue swelling in the right thigh. The bone is intact. (b) Eight days later there are signs of osteomyelitis with lucencies within the bone, periosteal reaction and a fracture of the upper shaft. The soft tissue swelling is extensive around the hip joint as is seen in septic arthritis. (c) Two weeks later there is extensive callus formation about the fracture. The soft tissue swelling has decreased. (d) In another 4 weeks the soft tissue swelling has cleared and there is remodelling of the callus.

Septic arthritis

In the neonate, the usual infective organisms are *Streptococcus pyogenes*, *Staphylococcus aureus* and *Haemophilus influenzae*. The infection affects the lower extremity with the hip and knee in 90%. The usual presentation is pain and pseudoparalysis. The affected area is warm and swollen and the infant usually presents a septic clinical picture.

The white cell count and C-reactive protein concentration are elevated. Aspiration of the joint for culture is usually undertaken. Initially radiographs are frequently normal. Sequelae of septic arthritis include growth disturbances, chronic degenerative arthritis and osteonecrosis. Figure 7.28 is a series of films showing the changes of osteomyelitis and septic arthritis.

Involvement in congenital infections

The incidence of congenital infection in the fetus and newborn infant is high, 0.5–2.5%. The most common causes are rubella virus, cytomegalovirus (CMV), toxoplasmosis and more rarely treponemal infections. Some infants are identified in the neonatal period because of intrauterine growth retardation, central nervous system symptoms and other organ system involvement – hepatomegaly, splenomegaly, pneumonia, bone lesions or anaemia. However, many of these infections are asymptomatic and a high index of suspicion is required.

Radiological signs of congenital infection are shown in Figure 7.29–7.32.

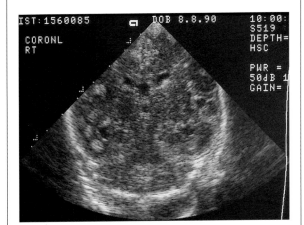

Fig. 7.29 US of the head showing scattered, patchy echogenic calcifications in the parenchyma consistent with toxoplasmosis.

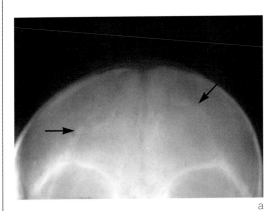

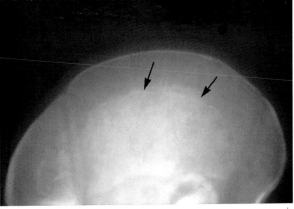

Fig. 7.30 Frontal (a) and lateral (b) skull X-rays with periventricular calcifications seen in congenital cytomegalovirus infection (arrows).

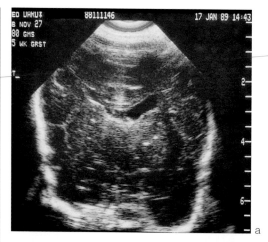

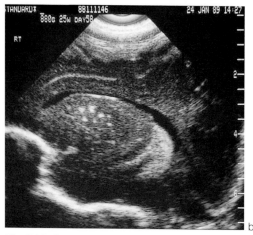

Fig. 7.31 Coronal (a) and sagittal (b) views from a cranial ultrasound scan of the head in a neonate with a CMV infection. There are multiple tiny echogenicities representing calcifications within the brain parenchyma.

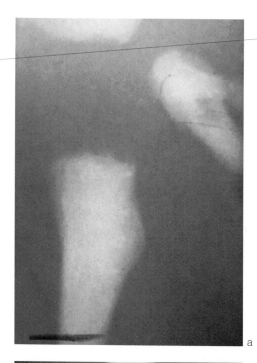

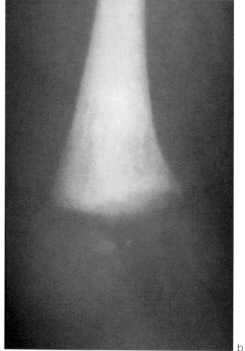

Fig. 7.32 Plain film views of the upper (a) and lower (b) end of the femur of a neonate with CMV infection. Irregular, linear lucencies are seen ('celery stalks').

Trauma

During delivery, especially of a large fetus, fractures of the clavicle can occur (Fig. 7.33). Crepitus may be felt over the fracture. The infant also needs to be evaluated for signs of brachial plexus nerve injury, as this may coexist.

Cranial injury (Fig. 7.34) can also occur following traumatic delivery. Usually they require no further treatment; however a neurosurgical opinion should be sought for depressed fractures.

References

Foster B K 1995 Initial screening and diagnosis of and referral for developmental dysplasia of the hip. Current Opinion in Pediatrics 7(1): 80–82.

Jones K I 1997 Smith's Recognizable patterns of human malformation, 5th edn. Saunders, Philadelphia

Silverman F N, Kuhn J P (eds) 1993 Caffey's Pediatric X-ray diagnosis, 9th edn. Mosby, St Louis

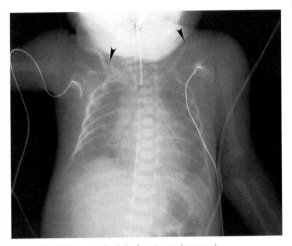

Fig. 7.33 Bilateral clavicle fractures (arrows).

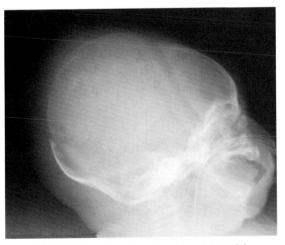

Fig. 7.34 Skull X-ray showing extensive extracranial tissue swelling and suture diastasis. CT showed subgaleal haemorrhage.

BONE

CHAPTER 8

Misplaced tubes and lines

Gerald Gill

Haresh Kirpalani

John Mernagh

Perhaps the most frequent reason for taking X-rays in the early days of life of the extremely preterm infant is to ensure correct positioning of tubes and lines. These include indwelling intravenous and intraarterial lines, endotracheal tubes, and drainage tubes including nasogastric and pneumothorax tubes. This chapter contains a series of images showing common and not-so-common problems encountered in placing lines and tubes.

ENDOTRACHEAL TUBE MANAGEMENT

Clinical signs are used to determine the initial placement of the endotracheal tube (ETT): these are chest wall movement, breath sounds and oxygen saturation. This procedure can be assisted by using published guidelines (Coldiron, 1968). Auscultation of the chest in newborns is unreliable except for very experienced clinicians, who still must obtain confirmation.

The ideal position is to place the tube with the tip between 0.5 cm above the carina and below the body of T1, with the head midline and in a neutral position. Unfortunately this positioning is achieved infrequently, especially in the middle of the night! When the head is flexed the ETT is brought higher, and conversely when the head is extended the ETT is lower. This is why positioning of the head is important and should be standardized for the examination.

Significant complications can result from malplacement, therefore a chest X-ray is mandatory. When malposition is noted, a more precise positioning should be made. Measurements on CXR can guide this repositioning (see below). The examples shown in Figures 8.1 and 8.2 illustrate some problems of malplacement of ETT.

Figure 8.3 shows another problem of malplacement that could not be predicted by the standard AP film. A lateral film would have shown that the ETT was posterior to the trachea. Admittedly this is a far rarer problem.

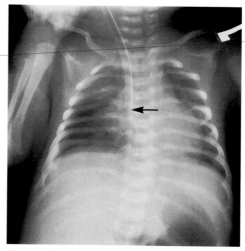

Fig. 8.1 Endotracheal tube with its tip in the right main bronchus (arrow). Here the left lung is not being well ventilated. On occasion, the pattern of air trapping leads to overdistension of the lung.

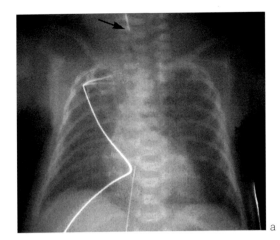

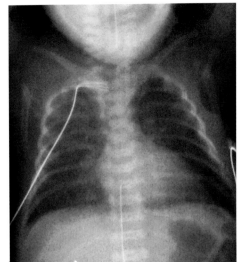

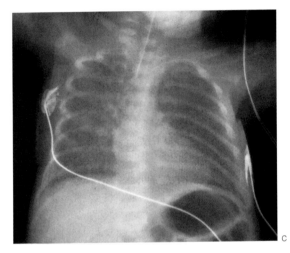

Fig. 8.2 On the initial film (a) the ETT tip is very high, at about the C5–6 vertebrae level (arrow). It should be advanced about 1.5 cm to reach the ideal position. However, it was advanced only 0.5 cm and on the next film (b) it is still high. A further 1 cm advancement (c) brings it to the T2 vertebra level, which is in the ideal range.

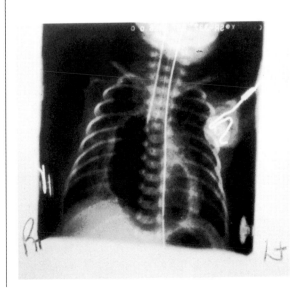

Fig. 8.3 An unusual cause of pneumomediastinum, from tracheal rupture proved at postmortem. In preterm infants the posterior constrictor muscles of the pharynx are often deficient or weak. This allows possible posterior penetration of the endotracheal tube into the mediastinum. In addition, the trachea is fragile and may be traumatized below the larynx.

NASOGASTRIC TUBE PLACEMENT

Placement of the nasogastric (NG) tube, and checking its position by listening for injected air over the abdomen is a frequent clinical manoeuvre. However, ensuring the correct placement of the NG tube does necessitate an abdominal X-ray (Fig. 8.4). A common misplacement is for the tube to be too high. If feeding is then commenced, the risk of pulmonary aspiration is great. In cases where the placement is beyond the stomach, the clinical presentation may be that of repeated large amounts of bilious drainage. Perforation may infrequently occur, as shown in Figures 8.5 and 8.6. The infant shown in Figure 8.6 was born at 26 weeks gestational age and was X-rayed aged 7 days for increased ventilation requirements. A nasogastric tube had been placed without apparent difficulty 12 hours previously. Oesophageal perforation was diagnosed. The tube was removed and the infant treated with antibiotics for 10 days, amazingly without further short-term or long-term sequelae.

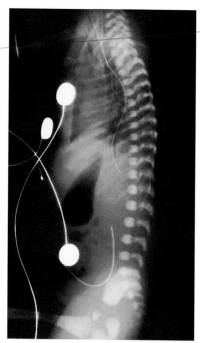

Fig. 8.5 Lateral view of the chest and abdomen showing an NG tube with the tip turning posteriorly away from the stomach. It has perforated, either from the pharynx into the mediastinum or into the abdomen at the gastrooesophageal junction. There is air tracking into the upper mediastinum, so the perforation is probably high.

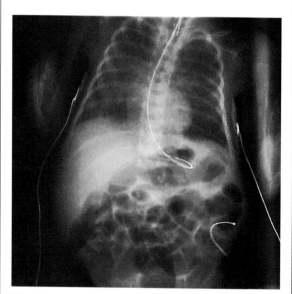

Fig. 8.4 An AP film of the chest with a correctly placed NG tube.

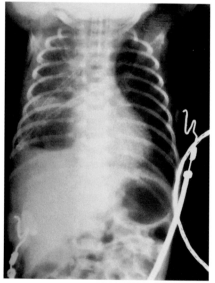

Fig. 8.6 Nasogastric tube perforation. The NG tube is seen to extend down the mediastinum parallel to the ETT and then veer to the right costophrenic angle, where it abruptly turns back with its tip at the mediastinum. There is some pleural fluid seen mainly in the minor fissure. This tube has perforated into the mediastinum and then into the right pleural space.

UMBILICAL CATHETERIZATION

The usual portals of entry for venous and arterial access in the emergency treatment of newborns are described below.

Arterial access

Recommendations from randomized trials are that placement should be high or low – that is to say either above T6 or at L3–5, i.e. presumably below the renal arteries (Figs 8.7, 8.8). Metaanalysis of small trials shows benefit (as assessed by rate of thrombus associated with the catheter) from a high position, which however, is balanced by a tendency to a higher rate of both necrotizing enterocolitis and possibly intraventricular haemorrhage in high positions (Schick et al 1989; see metaanalysis by Barrington). Other complications of placing such catheters include thrombus, vasospasm and renal hypertension.

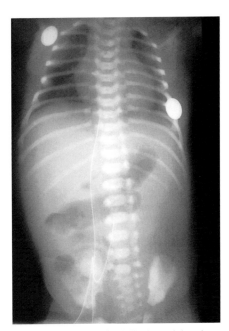

Fig. 8.7 Correct position of unbilical arterial and venous lines (AP view).

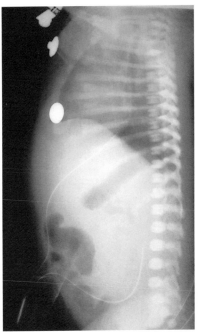

Fig. 8.8 Correct position of unbilical arterial and venous lines (lateral view).

Venous access

Complications include thrombus of the portal system and inferior vena cava (IVC), although this is thought to be rare.

Depth of insertion

Guidelines exist for depth of insertion of catheters into both unbilical arteries and veins (Dunn 1992). As for ETT, placement should be followed by radiological confirmation of position. Figure 8.9 shows graphs for umbilical artery and vein placement based on the length from shoulder to umbilicus. Understanding the correct placement of the lines requires some knowledge of the anatomy of the fetal and neonatal circulation (Fig. 8.10).

Figures 8.7 and 8.8 are anteroposterior (AP) and lateral films showing the correct position of umbilical arterial and venous lines. On the AP film the venous line should be to the right of the midline. The arterial line is seen to curve inferiorly, then superiorly, ending with its tip at or to the left of the midline. On the lateral film the arterial line is again seen to curve inferiorly then superiorly, posterior to the venous line. Sometimes legitimate confusion exists on an AP view as to whether the line is indeed a venous or an arterial line. The lateral film will sort out such confusions, as it will show the arterial line posteriorly adjacent to the spine, while the venous line will be seen anterior and then dipping posteriorly.

Figures 8.11–8.18 illustrate a variety of catheter placement problems, explained in the legends.

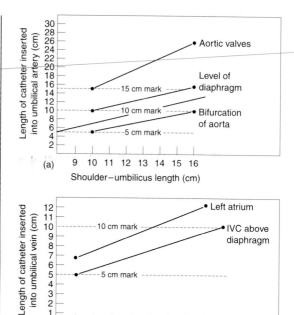

Fig. 8.9 Guide to catheterization of (a) umbilical artery and (b) umbilical vein, using an end-hole catheter marked at 5 cm, 10 cm and 15 cm from the tip (total length 38 cm). From Dunn (1975).

Fig. 8.10 The postnatal circulation and the path of the umbilical vasculature. (Modified from Moore 1982.) Dark shading indicates oxygenated or arterial blood; light shading indicates deoxygenated or venous blood. Not shown in the figure is the path from the umbilicus to the placenta; emerging from the skin the umbilical vessels in the fetus continue into the placenta, where, in-utero, the umbilical vein provides oxygenated blood from the placenta to the fetus, and the umbilical arteries are returning the deoxygenated blood to the placenta. The ductus venosus is shown, by which most of the blood supply 'bypasses' the lungs. The ductus venosus which, in-utero, bypasses the liver, so that the most oxygenated blood can be tracked to the upper extremities. Ideally, the umbilical venous catheter should cannulate the ductus venosus and enters the supra-diaphragmatic portion of the vena cava. It can be seen that the umbilical artery enters the internal iliac artery and then into the common iliac and then should move in an upward direction – this path can be seen on the films and helps to distinguish radiologically which vessels have been cannulated.

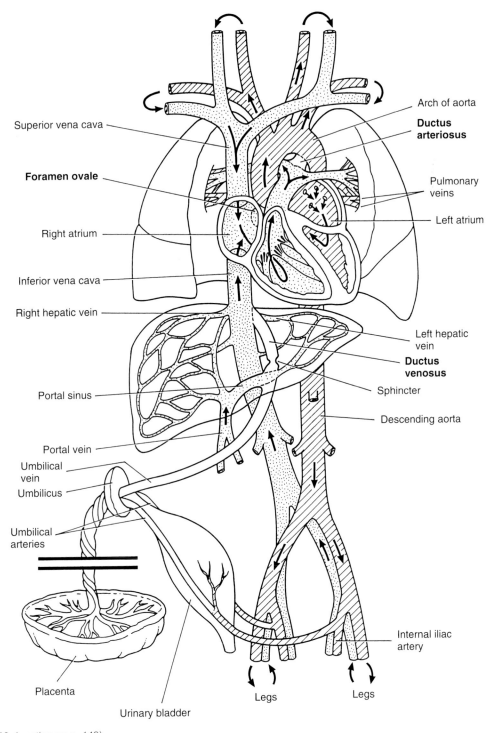

Superior vena cava

Foramen ovale

Right atrium

Inferior vena cava

Right hepatic vein

Portal sinus

Portal vein

Umbilical vein

Umbilicus

Umbilical arteries

Placenta

Urinary bladder

Arch of aorta

Ductus arteriosus

Pulmonary veins

Left atrium

Left hepatic vein

Ductus venosus

Sphincter

Descending aorta

Internal iliac artery

Legs

Legs

Fig. 8.10 (caption on p. 148)

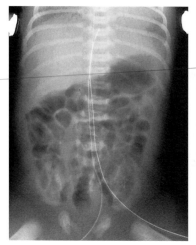

Fig. 8.11 Neonate with two umbilical venous lines instead of one venous and one arterial line. An arterial line would extend down the umbilical artery to the iliac artery before turning up into the aorta.

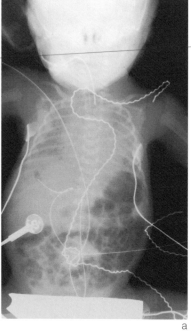

a

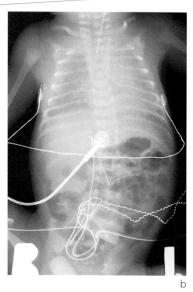

b

Fig. 8.12 Two neonates with malpositioned umbilical venous lines. (a) The line goes up from the umbilical vein to the portal vein. There is a gas density in the line near its tip. Possible causes: (1) air embolus, (2) focal necrosis, (3) necrotizing enterocolitis. (b) The line is placed up the umbilical vein and down the portal vein. The tip is probably in the superior mesenteric vein.

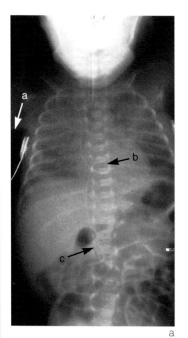

a

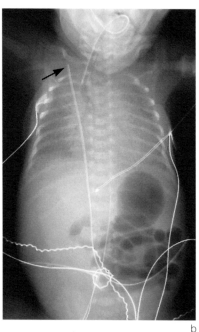

b

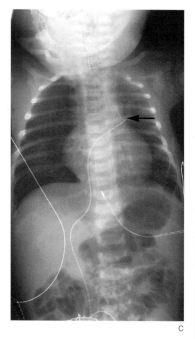

c

Fig. 8.13 Neonates with malpositioned venous lines. (a) From the right antecubital vein (arrow a), the line crosses the superior vena cava to the right atrium where it is coiled (arrow b), and then to the inferior vena cava (arrow c). (b) Umbilical venous line with the tip in the superior vena cava to the right jugular vein. (c) Venous line crossing the right atrium, foramen ovale and left atrium with its tip in a left pulmonary vein. Arrows show tip of line.

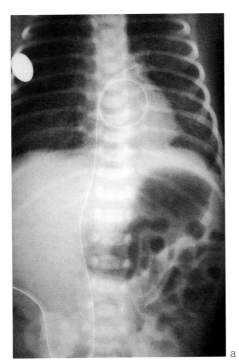
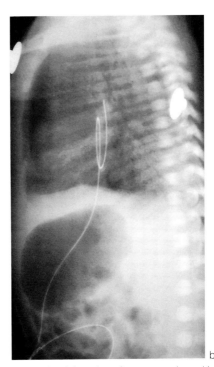

Fig. 8.14 AP (a) and lateral (b) films showing a venous line which crosses the right atrium, foramen ovale and is curled in the left atrium (note the posterior position of the loop as seen on the lateral film).

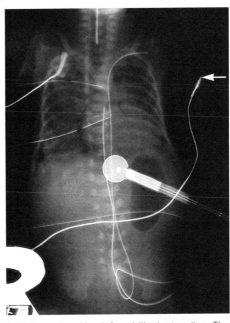

Fig. 8.15 Neonate with a left umbilical artery line. The line goes up the aorta and enters the left subclavian artery. Arrow shows tip of line.

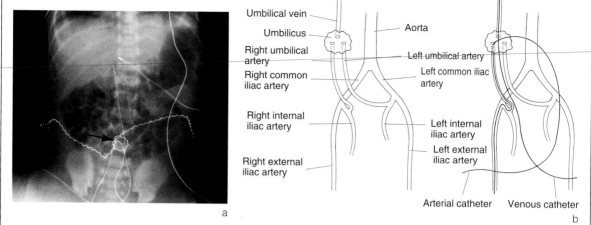

a
b

Fig. 8.16 (a) Neonate with a right umbilical artery line. The line goes down the right umbilical artery, to the right internal iliac artery, to the right external iliac artery and then down the right common femoral artery. Arrow denotes umbilicus.
(b) Line diagram illustrating the position of the right umbilical artery line on Fig. 8.16a. Note diagram's 'umbilicus' is offset.

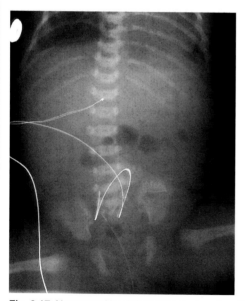

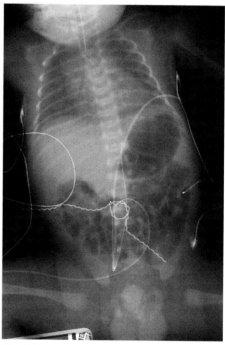

Fig. 8.17 Neonate with a left umbilical artery line. The line goes down the left umbilical artery to the left common iliac artery, then crosses via the aorta to the right common iliac artery and then to the right umbilical artery.

Fig. 8.18 Neonate with two right umbilical artery lines instead of one venous and one arterial line.

References

Barrington K Metaanalysis on umbilical artery catheters: catheter position. At: http://silk.nih.gov/silk/cochrane/Barring 1/ Barring1.htm

Coldiron J S 1968 Estimation of NT tube length in neonates. Pediatrics 41: 825

Dunn P M, Modified by Llewellyn M A 1975 In: Swyer P R (ed.) The intensive care of the newly born. Karger, Basel

Moore K L 1982 The developing human, 3rd edn. Saunders, Philadelphia

Schick J B, Beck A L, DeSilva H N 1989 UAC position and IVH. Journal of Perinatology 9: 382–385

CHAPTER 9

Prenatal ultrasonography

Pat Mohide
Haresh Kirpalani
John Mernagh

Ultrasonography has revolutionized modern obstetrics. It is the only tool that allows for the complete physical examination of the fetus. It has been applied to many screening, diagnostic and therapeutic situations and has shown its greatest usefulness in screening for fetal anomalies.

WHO SHOULD BE SCREENED?

Most women who deliver fetuses with anomalies do *not* have identified risk factors such as drug or alcohol use, infections or a family history. To be effective, screening *must* therefore be applied to healthy women without known risks. Randomized clinical trials (RCTs) and population-based studies show that screening for fetal anomalies is highly effective when performed at 18–20 weeks of pregnancy. Some anomalies such as anencephaly can be detected as early as 12 weeks. The same RCTs also show increased terminations of pregnancies with fetal anomalies, early diagnosis of twins at 20–26 weeks, reduced admissions of neonates to special care, fewer birthweights below 2500 g and few inductions of labour for 'post-dates' pregnancy (Neilson 1995). All these are clinically important outcomes. For example, missed twin pregnancy may have serious consequences.

ULTRASOUND AND 'FETAL HEALTH'

Obstetricians have long sought a method to detect the fetus in trouble in the third trimester who is at risk of intrauterine death, birth asphyxia, and newborn or later morbidity. The biophysical profile (an ultrasound scoring of fetal movement, tone, breathing movements and amniotic fluid volume combined with fetal heart rate monitoring) or fetal heart rate monitoring alone did appear to improve detection of such fetuses, but failed to show clinical benefit in two RCTs (Mohide & Keirse 1989). More promising is the recent development of Doppler evaluation of blood flow velocities in the umbilical artery. Eleven RCTs (excluding a twelfth badly flawed trial) of Doppler screening in high-risk pregnancies have

shown significant reductions in stillbirths, antepartum hospital admissions, elective delivery and induction of labour. Statistically non-significant trends to improvement were found for preterm birth, emergency caesarean section and neonatal death (Neilson & Alfirevic 1995).

ETHICAL ISSUES IN ULTRASOUND

Issues regarding termination

For some, the use of ultrasound to detect anomalies and increase the use of abortion is troublesome. Consent is not always fully informed in patients being sent for ultrasound scans where fetal anomalies may be detected. Some may not wish to know and face the difficult decisions which may follow. For patients who wish to adopt a course of termination following appropriate counselling, the earlier the diagnosis is made the easier the situation is. Different regulations apply in different countries.

Regulations concerning ultrasound

Despite the safe use of ultrasound since the early 1970s, continuing surveillance and evaluation by governments and professional bodies, regulations applied to the manufacture of ultrasound machines, and practice guidelines for the safe use of ultrasound, concerns are still expressed. Continued vigilance is still warranted, as basic scientific evidence suggests that high energy levels or prolonged continuous exposure to ultrasound energy have the potential to cause harm. Probably much more important is the potential for harm arising from missed diagnoses or false labelling. In these latter cases there may be a failure to implement available, appropriate clinical care, or conversely risky interventions may be applied without clinical benefit.

Gender

Gender identification is a common patient request but occasional incidents have occurred where patients have gone on to request abortion, usually of a female fetus. This has led some ultrasonographers to refuse to identify gender in early pregnancy (< 24 weeks), unless there is a medical indication.

Non-medical issues

Some ultrasound scans appear to be performed for non-medical indications such as curiosity, reassurance, gender identification and what some have called 'recreation'. Participation of publicly paid health workers in 'frivolous' medical procedures concerns many. This must be balanced by a recognition that pregnancy is usually a healthy state and not a disease, and that ultrasound investigations may have positive effects on maternal attachment and reduce the use of cigarettes and alcohol.

Precision

Ultrasonography is still not 100% precise in the detection of abnormality. The failure to detect represents a lost opportunity for effective treatment. More frequent and worrisome is the still unacceptably high rate of false-positive diagnosis of placenta praevia, suspect fetal anomalies, oligo- and polyhydramnios and fetal compromise, leading to unnecessary anxiety and sometimes inappropriate clinical action.

THE TEAM APPROACH

Prenatal care is provided routinely by family physicians, midwives, obstetricians and nurses. When maternal complications develop, consultation and collaboration should occur with maternal-fetal medicine specialists, internists, haematologists, thrombosis teams, immunologists and endocrinologists. When fetal problems are identified, it is also appropriate to consult and share care with neonatologists, paediatric surgeons, neurosurgeons, neurologists, developmental paediatricians, geneticists and social workers. A major focus of the management of the mother carrying a fetus with anomalies is counselling to ensure full information is conveyed to the patient. Only on this basis can any sensible decision be made. Such full information-giving can then result in a sensible clinical decision, which

accounts for expressed parental preferences. Maternal and fetal patients are often referred as outpatients or inpatients to regional programmes in perinatal care, genetics and prenatal diagnosis. Where there are specialized needs for care and assessment in labour, at birth and during newborn care, delivery at a regional centre may be planned, for example in cases of serious congenital heart defects. A final and complete diagnosis may not be possible in utero and often awaits careful and detailed evaluation of the newborn.

SPINA BIFIDA

Spina bifida is failure of neural tube closure at 18–23 days from conception. This has potentially serious long-term sequelae which include major surgical requirements.

Clinical features

The lesion is usually lumbosacral, but can occur in cervical and thoracic regions. It is often associated with posterior displacement of the cerebellum, obliteration of the cisterna magna (Arnold–Chiari type 2) and hydrocephalus. Kyphosis, scoliosis and abnormal vertebral elements are common. The higher the lesion, the worse the neurological prognosis may be.

Presentation

Spina bifida is most frequently detected in prenatal ultrasound scans at 16–20 weeks and by maternal serum screening at 15 weeks for elevated levels of alphafetoprotein (AFP).

Management

Referral to and delivery in a regional perinatal centre is necessary. Antenatal consultations should be arranged with a neonatologist and a paediatric neurosurgeon. The fetus should be monitored for hydrocephalus. The neonatal team should be present at delivery. Caesarean section may be considered for breech presentation in labour.

Ultrasonographic appearance

The characteristic US signs of spina bifida are shown in Figures 9.1–9.4.

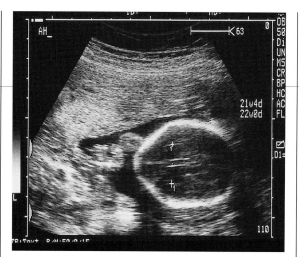

Fig. 9.1 Spina bifida. 'Lemon' sign, indicating indentation of anterior cranial vault.

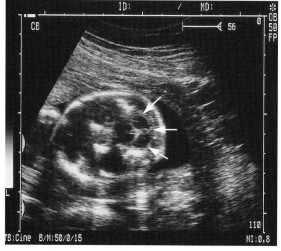

Fig. 9.2 Spina bifida. 'Banana' sign, indicating bowing of the cerebellum and its vermis (see arrows).

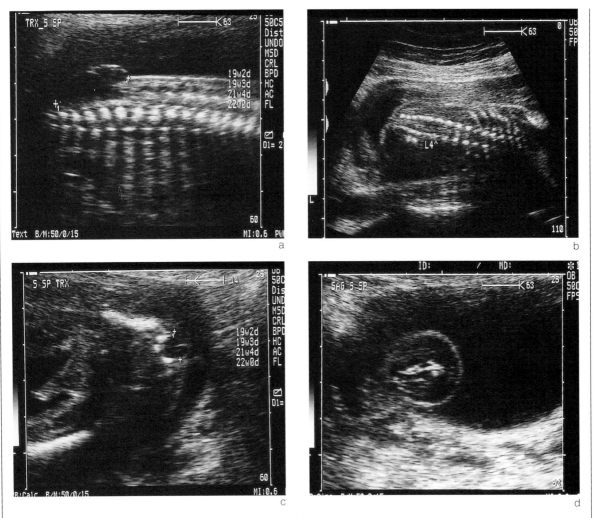

Fig. 9.3 Lumbosacral meningomyelocele. (a) Sagittal view. (b) Coronal view of the spine showing splaying of lumbosacral elements. (c) Axial (transverse) view of the spine showing splaying of vertebral arches. (d) Coronal view of the meningomyocele showing neural elements within it.

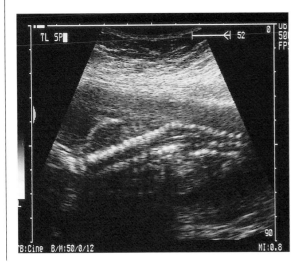

Fig. 9.4 Kyphoscoliosis – note the severe angulation and disorganization of spine in association with a thoracolumbar spina bifida.

INTRAUTERINE GROWTH RETARDATION

Intrauterine growth retardation (IUGR) is the severe slowing or absence of fetal growth in utero resulting in low birthweight for gestational age (usually below the 2.5 percentile).

Clinical features

There is a wide clinical spectrum with a diverse aetiology. There are three main groups:

- genetic predisposition to smallness (physiological)
- intrinsic fetal problem (e.g. trisomy)
- extrinsic compromise of uteroplacental supply (e.g. toxaemia, chronic abruption, lupus).

Presentation

The condition is usually recognized because the uterus is clinically 'small for dates' or because of maternal risk factors (e.g. proteinuric hypertension). Most common ultrasound findings are poor growth of measured parameters such as abdominal circumference, biparietal diameter, lower than expected estimates of fetal weight, oligohydramnios, assessed qualitatively or by measurement (four-quadrant amniotic fluid index or deepest pocket, Fig. 9.5), and reduced, absent, or reversed umbilical artery end-diastolic velocities (Figs 9.6 and 9.7).

Management

Serial ultrasound scans are required every 2 weeks to assess growth. Weekly or more frequent ultrasound scans are needed for biophysical and Doppler flow assessments. Amniocentesis may be considered for early-onset IUGR. Investigations and treatment of maternal disease (e.g. hypertension, diabetes) are needed, as are antenatal consultations with neonatology and internal medicine specialists, when relevant. Caesarean section should be performed where there are signs of fetal distress, and the neonatal team should be present at the delivery.

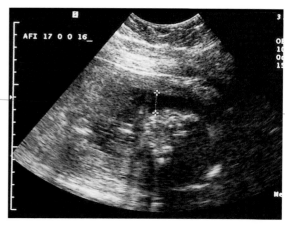

Fig. 9.5 Oligohydramnios: the deepest pocket is measured in four quadrants of the amniotic sac. The total in this case is 33 mm.

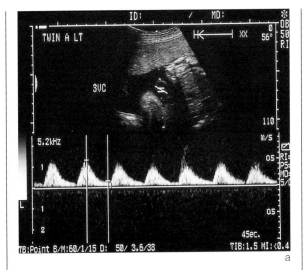

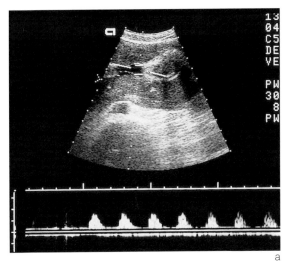

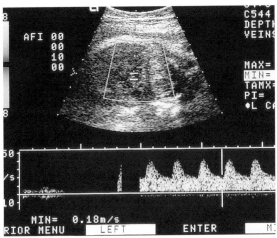

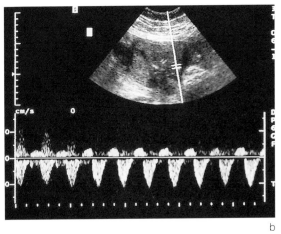

Fig. 9.6 Umbilical artery with reduced end-diastolic flow. (a) This suggests increased placental vascular resistance. (b) Middle cerebral artery showing enhanced end-diastolic flow. This suggests a physiological response to hypoxia.

Fig. 9.7 Umbilical artery showing absent end-diastolic flow. (a) This suggests high placental vascular resistance and implies fetal compromise. (b) Umbilical artery showing reversed end-diastolic flow.

HYDROCEPHALUS

Hydrocephalus is defined as dilatation of the cerebral ventricles.

Clinical features

Hydrocephalus is usually detected any time from 18 weeks of gestation onward. It is often associated with spina bifida. There are many other associations including other intracranial pathology, skeletal dysplasias, multiple anomaly syndromes and chromosomal anomalies.

Presentation

Most commonly hydrocephalus is found at the standard 18–20 week ultrasound anomaly screen or as a surprise finding in later pregnancy ultrasound scans.

Management

Referral to and delivery in a regional perinatal centre is necessary. Antenatal consultations with neonatology, paediatric neurosurgery and genetics specialists should be arranged where appropriate. Caesarean section is only required for obstetrical indications.

Ultrasonographic appearance

The characteristic findings of hydrocephalus are shown in Figures 9.8–9.10.

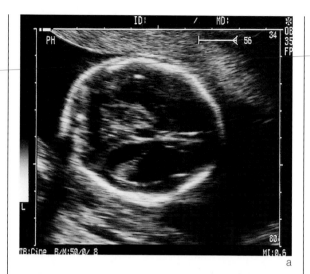

a

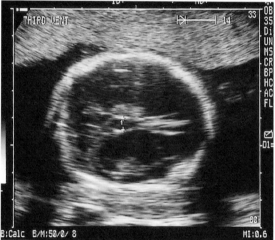

b

Fig. 9.8 Hydrocephalus. Axial (transverse) view of dilated lateral ventricles. (a) Note the associated 'dangling choroid plexus'. (b) A prominent third ventricle is noted in the midline between the thalami.

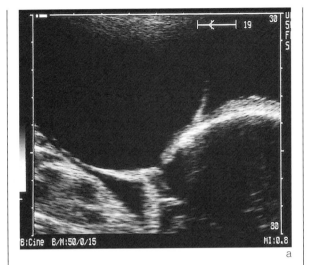

a

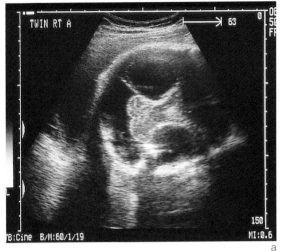

a

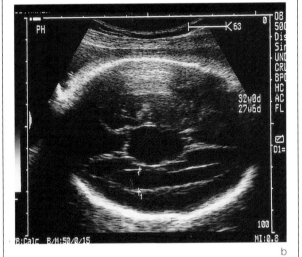

b

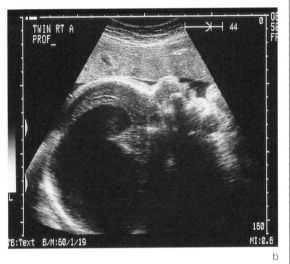

b

Fig. 9.9 Hydrocephalus associated with posterior fossa cyst and a posterior encephalocele. (a) Posterior encephalocele communicating through a small defect in the occipital bone. (b) Dilated lateral and third ventricles and a posterior fossa cyst (note: cerebellum was present at a lower level).

Fig. 9.10 Severe hydrocephalus in twins. (a) Note marked dilatation of both lateral ventricles, posterior fossa cyst and small cerebellum. (b) Sagittal view of the same case with posterior horns more dilated than anterior. The parents were first cousins.

OMPHALOCELE

Omphalocele is the herniation of abdominal contents into the base of the umbilical cord (after 12 weeks gestation) owing to a midline defect of the anterior abdominal wall secondary to failure of the lateral body folds to fuse during weeks 3–4 of gestation. Physiological herniation of the gut at 8–12 weeks is a normal finding.

Clinical features

Presentation

Omphalocele is most frequently detected by prenatal ultrasonography. It may also be detected by elevation of maternal serum AFP levels at 15–20 weeks (due to leakage of AFP across the sac membrane into amniotic fluid). It is sometimes associated with ascites, but bowel obstruction is uncommon. Omphalocele is frequently associated with other malformations (75%) and chromosomal anomalies (45%): common associations are heart, genitourinary and intestinal (atresias) anomalies.

Management

Referral to and delivery at a regional perinatal centre is necessary. Antenatal consultations should be arranged with neonatologist and a paediatric surgeon. Caesarean section is indicated for obstetrical reasons only. The neonatal team should be present at delivery.

Ultrasonographic appearance

The midline defect may involve the entire ventral abdominal wall. The cord inserts at the apex of the defect. There is herniation of abdominal viscera at the base of the umbilical cord including liver (30%) with a covering peritoneal/amniotic membrane (Figs 9.11, 9.12). Polyhydramnios may be present and there is a high incidence of associated anomalies (45–70%): chromosomal, genitourinary, cardiac and neural tube defects, IUGR, Beckwith–Wiedemann syndrome and gastrointestinal tract abnormalities. The mortality rate is 30–55% owing to associated abnormalities.

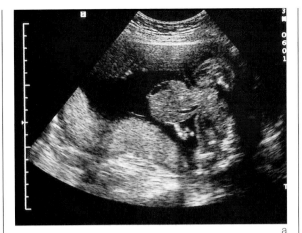

a

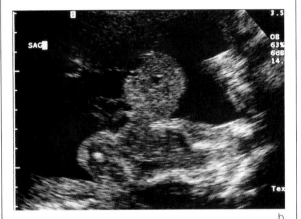

b

Fig. 9.11 Omphalocele with bowel and liver. The sac is surrounded by a thin membrane. (a) There is no evidence of dilatation of bowel within the defect. (Note: the fetus is upside down.) (b) The same sac showing cord insertion into the sac.

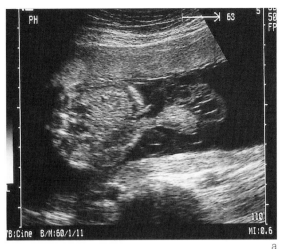

a

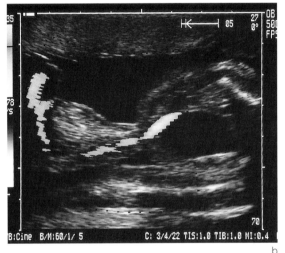

b

Fig. 9.12 A small omphalocele identified at 20 weeks in an otherwise normal fetus. (a) Distal to the omphalocele is a 'false knot' in the cord. Postnatal surgery was a complete success. (b) Umbilical vessels are demonstrated with colour Doppler to pass beside the small hernial sac.

GASTROSCHISIS

Gastroschisis is a paraumbilical fusion defect usually on the right side secondary to premature interruption of the right omphalomesenteric artery or abnormal involution of the right umbilical vein at 5 weeks of gestational age.

Ultrasonographic findings (Figs 9.13, 9.14) include normal insertion of umbilical cord, and normal or thickened freely floating bowel loops outside the fetal abdomen with lack of peritoneal covering. The defect is usually on the right side of the cord insertion. There is no fetal ascites.

Polyhydramnios may be present. Bowel obstruction or perforation may be a complication. The incidence of associated anomalies is 5%.

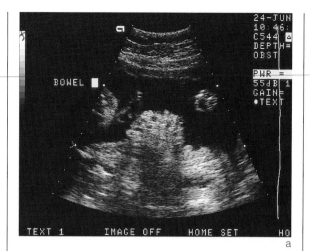

a

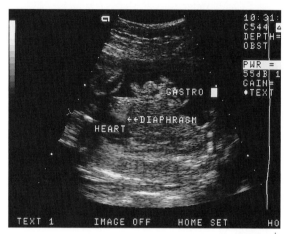

b

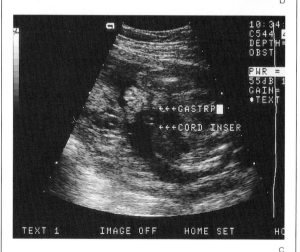

c

Fig. 9.13 Gastroschisis. Three views (a–c) from a prenatal US scan showing a loop of non-dilated bowel protruding from a defect in the abdominal wall to the right of the insertion of the umbilical cord.

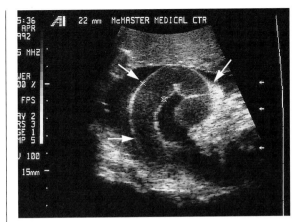

Fig. 9.14 Gastroschisis. This patient has a loop of fluid-filled, dilated bowel (see arrows) protruding from the abdominal wall defect.

References

Mohide P T, Keirse M J N C 1989 Biophysical assessment of fetal well-being in effective care. In: Pregnancy and childbirth, vol. 1, pp 477–492. Oxford University Press

Neilson J P 1995 Routine ultrasound in early pregnancy (revised 5 December 1994). In: Keirse M J N C, Renfrew M J, Neilson J P, Crowther C (eds) Pregnancy and childbirth module. Cochrane Database of Systemic Reviews (database on disk and CD-ROM). The Cochrane Collaboration; issue 2. Oxford, Update Software, available from BMJ Publishing Group, London

Neilson J P, Alfirevic Z 1995 Doppler ultrasound in high risk pregnancies (revised 23 July 1995). In: Keirse M J N C, Renfrew M J, Neilson J P, Crowther C (eds) Pregnancy and childbirth module. Cochrane Database of Systemic Reviews (database on disk and CD-ROM). The Cochrane Collaboration, issue 2. Oxford, Update Software, available from BMJ Publishing Group, London.

Index